Self-Expression through Art and Drumming

Self-Expression
through **Art**
and **Drumming**

*A Facilitator's Guide to Using
Art Therapy to Enhance Drum Circles*

JEN MANK

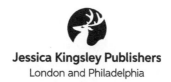

Jessica Kingsley Publishers
London and Philadelphia

First published in Great Britain in 2021 by Jessica Kingsley Publishers
An Hachette Company

1

Copyright © Jen Mank 2021

Front cover image source: Jen Mank

A CIP catalogue record for this title is available from the
British Library and the Library of Congress

ISBN 978 1 78592 715 7
eISBN 978 1 78450 310 9

Printed and bound in the United Stated by Integrated Books International

Jessica Kingsley Publishers' policy is to use papers that are natural,
renewable and recyclable products and made from wood grown in
sustainable forests. The logging and manufacturing processes are expected
to conform to the environmental regulations of the country of origin.

Jessica Kingsley Publishers
Carmelite House
50 Victoria Embankment
London EC4Y 0DZ

www.jkp.com

I dedicate this work to my husband, Dick, who spent countless hours helping with developing the working design of the self-ascribed drums in this book. His ingenuity and diligence made the final design possible. I would also like to thank Arthur Hull and Christine Stevens for their contagious love of music and drumming that has propelled me on this journey of music, love and belonging.

Acknowledgments

I would like to thank Nicholas Sager for all his help and support in encouraging me to explore the intersection of art therapy and music therapy. I am grateful to my art therapy professors who taught me to use creativity to gain a greater understanding of self and others through the arts. Kathy Quain and Arthur Hull offered community in the form of drum circles and drum circle facilitation education. The education in drum circle facilitation continued with Mary Knish and Christine Stevens. All along the way, the drum circle community welcomed me and provided unconditional support. I also want to extend that welcoming and sense of belonging to others through written form.

Everyone at Jessica Kingsley Publishers provided support to create a book in which others can continue the work and community building that drum circles provide. The patience, support and direction provided by Jane Evans, Simeon Hance and Claire Robinson was, and still is, greatly appreciated. This book would still be in the dreaming phase without the encouragement and support provided by all the staff at Jessica Kingsley Publishers.

Throughout my participation, research and education in drum circles I have been welcomed and offered acceptance and education to grow and develop as a drummer, drum circle facilitator, researcher, therapist and community member, and as an individual. I want to acknowledge and offer my gratitude to all the drummers and drum circle facilitators that have welcomed me into the drum circle community. I hope this book continues all the efforts you began before me and will aid those that continue the work and efforts to bring people together in peace and community through drumming.

This book is based on the papers written, research conducted and dissertation completed in order to achieve my PhD in art therapy.

Contents

Introduction 11
Expressive Therapies Continuum   12
Object relations theory   13
Conclusion   17

1. Art Therapy 19
Historical roots   19
Art and humans   21
Art making with the art therapy process   22
Neuroscience and art therapy   24
Expressive Therapies Continuum   26
Art processing and the Expressive Therapies Continuum   31
Brain structures and the ETC   32
Neuroplasticity   34
Conclusion   36

2. Psychodynamic Theory 37
Freud   37
Psychodynamic theory and art therapy   39
Transference and countertransference   40
Sublimation and art therapy   42
Sublimation and drumming   43
Object relations theory   44
Object relations theory and art therapy   48
Object relations theory and drumming   50
Attachment theory   51

Mirroring, attachment and neurological development   53

Attachment theory and drumming   56

Conclusion   57

3. Signs and Symbols   58

Symbols and culture   61

Dream imagery   62

Archetypes   62

Connection to symbols   63

Symbolic form within art therapy   65

Symbols, drum making and drumming   65

Conclusion   66

4. Music and Music Therapy.   67

Identity and the expressive arts   69

Music and mental health   71

Music therapy   72

Drumming and shamanic trances   74

Creativity   76

Improvisation   77

Drum circles   78

Conclusion   81

5. Drum History and Drum Making   82

Drumming and spirituality   82

Rhythm   84

Gender and drumming   84

Personal drum making history   85

Creating the symbol of self   104

Conclusion   107

6. Leading a Drum Circle   109

Structure of a drum circle   109

Drum circle facilitation   111

Role of the facilitator   112

Therapeutic drum circle etiquette   114

How to play a djembe or tubano drum   115

Therapeutic drum circle warm ups   116

Drum circle directives   120
Developing reciprocal relationships within the drum circle
environment   126
Facilitating the group   128
Assessment and attunement within the drum circle   128
The Expressive Therapies Continuum and drumming   129
Feedback   136
Reentry into drumming   137
Closing the drum circle session   138
Conclusion   139

Conclusion **140**

References *145*

Index *152*

Introduction

The expressive arts of art therapy and drumming offer therapeutic benefits that can include therapeutic growth and healing while creating attachments and a sense of belonging between members of the drum circle (Hull 2006; Mank 2019; Stevens 2017). The benefits of music playing and listening have been shown to benefit the individual through improvement of mood, shaping identity, and providing meaning in life (Darnley-Smith & Patey 2003; Semenza 2018; Wanjala & Kebaya 2016). However, without the therapeutic guidance of a trained music therapist, the experience cannot be described as music therapy (AMTA 2019).

Art making has potential for therapeutic growth and healing while building mastery (AATA 2020; Archibald *et al.* 2010). Art making and art therapy include sensory-based acquisition of information and knowledge that act to stimulate and engage the brain and the body in ways that verbal language cannot (AATA 2020). The arts provide alternative approaches to resolve problems, improve interpersonal skill sets, address and manage stress, and establish self-awareness and insight. In order for art making to be art therapy, one must be under the therapeutic care and guidance of a trained art therapist (AATA 2020).

This book aims to provide information pertaining to art and music therapy and the psychological theories that guide the therapist in providing care to the client. The reader will not be an art or music therapist as a result of reading the chapters of this book. Nor will the drum circles or art making be considered therapy as a result of reading these chapters. However, if the reader is an art or music therapist then the chapters may provide useful information in the practice of art or music therapy when used within the context of a therapeutic alliance and within the appropriate scope of practice of the therapist. The reader may also gain an awareness of the role of a therapist, the need for a therapeutic environment, and the benefits of demonstrating an unconditional positive regard for participants while facilitating a therapeutic drum circle. Drum circle directives and drum making instructions are provided to assist in facilitating a drum circle. The following chapters describe the therapeutic nature of art and music in order to provide positive experiences of art and music making within the drum circle experience. The information provided pertaining to art therapy, music therapy, neurological frameworks and theory, and psychological theories acts to inform the reader about the functioning of the participant and offers ideas and methods to best facilitate the group in art and music making.

Within the therapeutic environment of the art studio and the drum circle, the therapist provides unconditional positive regard for the participants, demonstrates mirroring and models appropriate behavior in order to build neuroplasticity, improve self-esteem, form secure attachment, and create a sense of belonging among the members of the group (Hinz 2009; King 2016; Kossak 2015; Lusebrink 2004, 2016; Mank 2019). The role of the art therapist is multifaceted and includes providing support and acceptance of the client and the art, being present in the moment, and creating art with the client to ensure the possibility of therapeutic growth and change, all within a therapeutic alliance and environment (Allen 1995; Chapman 2014; Rogers 2007). Art therapy is founded in service and healing (Broderick 2011). The art making is the tool used to achieve recovery and wellbeing within the art therapy process and therapeutic alliance (Broderick 2011).

Expressive Therapies Continuum

The kinesthetic movement of art making along with mindfulness and visual processing of the art results in neurological changes within the brain (Hass-Cohen & Findlay 2015; Hinz 2009; Lusebrink 2004). Art therapy has been shown to have the ability to utilize alternative neural pathways within the brain, known as neuroplasticity, with the goal of improving wellbeing and creative functioning (Chapman 2014; Hinz 2009; King 2016; Lusebrink 2004, 2016).

The Expressive Therapies Continuum (ETC) is a theoretical, hierarchical framework that informs and allows the therapist to identify strengths and possible visual processing blockages in the client (Hinz 2009). The ETC provides a means for the therapist to identify and classify how a client processes information and stimuli, in order to best serve the client. The goal of the therapist is to assist the client to reach a balance within a level or between all levels of the ETC in order to function on a Creative level (Hinz 2009).

It should be noted that the ETC should only be used by a trained therapist when assessing a client or participant utilizing the creative arts.

Object relations theory

Object relations theory provides theoretical insight to the therapist pertaining to the attachment style and psychological functioning of the client (Goldenberg & Goldenberg 2008; Kramer 1972; Naumburg 1973; Rubin 1987). Drumming can act as a way to divert pathological impulses into socially acceptable behavior through sublimation (Kramer 1972; Rubin 1987). The symbolic language of art provides access to the unconscious and facilitates the release of inner fantasies, fears and conflicts (Naumburg 1973; Rubin 1987). Attachment styles reflect the first relationship between the child and the primary caregiver (Goldenberg & Goldenberg 2008). Winnicott (2005) believed that the nurturing environment between the primary caregiver and the child allowed the child to attach in a healthy manner. Within the therapeutic alliance and environment, therapeutic change is possible (Corey 1996; Goldenberg & Goldenberg 2008; Kramer 1972; Naumburg 1973; Rubin 1987). Behavior and the attachment styles of an individual are malleable through therapeutic intervention and the expressive arts (Gillath *et al.* 2009).

CASE VIGNETTE

A case vignette is offered to the reader to demonstrate the effectiveness and benefits of creating a self-ascribed drum and playing it for ten weeks within a therapeutic drum circle. Arisa (a pseudonym), was a Caucasian female in her early sixties when she agreed to participate in a research study for art and drumming (Mank 2019). She was highly educated, having acquired a Ph.D. in a scientific field, and she resided in Northern California. She had spent over 20 years as a stay-at-home mother caring for two children with special needs. During the pre-interview she described her role as being "a slave" to her family, but now she was in transition with a changing role. As a mother of two children with special needs, Arisa had previously felt that she could not be herself and had to care for her children and husband. Now that her children were no longer minors, Arisa was less involved in their lives and allowed them greater independence while still offering support and co-parenting with her husband, from whom she was now separated. She was currently focused on trying to find a new identity and way of life that provided enjoyment and a sense of wellbeing. She had previous musical experience, was comfortable making music and was interested in creating improvisational music within a therapeutic drum circle.

The research group started the research study with pre-interviews, played commercial drums for ten weeks, carried out a post-assessment, painted a symbol of self on a homemade drum, and then played that drum for four more sessions (Mank 2019). Prior to and after drumming, Arisa was assessed using the Geriatric Depression Scale,[1] the Purpose in Life Test[2] and the State Adult Attachment Measure.[3] Arisa's pre-intervention score on the Geriatric Depression Scale indicated she had mild depression, with a score of 16 points. She took the Purpose in Life test and scored

1   The Geriatric Depression Scale (GDS) is assessment that is self-administered and consists of 30 questions that require binary answers of yes or no (Kurlowicz 2002). Total scores in the range of 0–9 fall within the normal mood range. Scores of 10–19 indicate mild depression. Scores of 20–30 are indicative of severe depression (Kurlowicz 2002).
2   The Purpose in Life Test (PIL) is designed to assess an older adult's level of happiness, satisfaction with life and emotional stability (Schulenberg, Schnetzern & Buchanan 2011). The PIL is a self-administered assessment with 21 items and a Likert scale of 1–5, with 5 rated as the strongest positive answer. The total scores of the PIL range from 20–100. A total score that is less than or equal to 50 suggests a current lack of purpose or meaning in the participant's life (Crumbaugh & Maholick 1964). The PIL possesses a positive correlation with hope and life satisfaction (Schulenberg et al. 2011).
3   The State Adult Attachment Measure (SAAM) is an assessment designed to measure an older adult's current attachment state (Gillath et al. 2009). There are 21 items and three subscales for attachment states: secure, anxious and avoidant. It is self-administered and the participant is asked to rate the level of accuracy of statements to their current state of attachment on a 7-point Likert scale, ranging from 1 = strongly disagree to 7 = strongly agree. The assessment contains seven statements to measure avoidance (e.g. "I feel alone and yet don't feel like getting close to others"), seven statements measuring anxiety (e.g. "I feel a strong need to be unconditionally loved right now") and seven additional questions that measure secure attachment (e.g. "I feel loved") (Gillath et al. 2009).

    The avoidant attachment subscale measures an individual's reluctance to trust others and the propensity to concentrate on autonomy and independence. This subscale also measures reluctance or resistance to interpersonal intimacy with a drive to reduce or downplay personal emotions and emotional responses. The anxiety subscale discerns an individual's low evaluation of personal abilities and self-worth with a desire to display a strong need for "personal closeness, love and support, and constant worrying about being rejected or abandoned" (Gillath et al. 2009). Finally, the secure attachment subscale is a measure of an individual's personal sense of self-worth, comfort with intimacy, and faith in reciprocity by attachment figures (Gillath et al. 2009).

72 points. The State Adult Attachment Measure showed her highest scores fell within the anxious attachment subscale at 6.57. The secure attachment subscale score was 4.86 and the avoidant subscale was 1.

Arisa had a positive affect and made friends easily within the group. While she reported that she had held in the past the role of leader and no longer wished to be one, she often set the rhythm within the drumming group. She reported that through drumming she was able to "let the beast out!" Arisa preferred to play the drums with her hands and not a mallet, and to have the tactile sensation of "pounding on the drum." She smiled and conversed with the other members of the group and laughed throughout the sessions. She reported (and was observed) starting a drum rhythm and then responding to rhythms played by other members of the group. She stated that conversations occurred through rhythm and that rhythms were "passed back and forth" within the drum circle. Drumming was a way to communicate without verbalization and to connect to others through rhythm.

Arisa enjoyed going into the inner space of the drum circle and sitting in a chair to feel the sound vibrations from the drumming of the members of the group. She reported that the experience of physically experiencing the sound vibrations was akin to being supported, accepted and loved by the group. Arisa also described how her sense of belonging to the group increased after her first experience of entering the inner space of the drum circle.

Outside of the drum circle, Arisa began to teach knitting and crochet to some of the group members. She offered advice and information on various subjects to the members of the group. She helped with the dismantling of the drum circle and the loading of the drums into a car. Overall, she reported she was no longer a leader but rather a supporter of the group. However, she continued to lead within the drumming and to share her knowledge and skills with others.

Arisa's post-assessment scores showed improvement over the pre-assessment scores. Her scores on the Geriatric Depression Scale decreased by six points, making her score one point away from what the scale defines as a normal mood. Her Purpose in Life test score increased by six points to 78. Her State Adult Attachment scores showed changes as well. She scored 6.14 on the Anxious subscale, which was a decrease of 0.43. Her Avoidant subscale score stayed at 1. The Secure Attachment subscale increased from 4.86 to 5.57, indicating an increase of 0.71 and a possible increase in secure attachment. Just as important were her qualitative self-reports of happiness as a result of drumming and the sense of finding a different identity than that of a slave.

During the post-interview, Arisa stated that this point in her life was one in which she was carving out "me time." She was a drummer, a quilter and a mother, and she belonged to a drumming group, a book club and a quilting group. Although she wanted to allocate more time to making friends, traveling and having fun, she was still dedicated to being a mother. She prided herself in learning to say "no" and to prioritize herself in order to practice self-care. Arisa discussed being apprehensive about how she would relate to other participants of the drum group prior to drumming. During the post-interview, she stated that she was surprised at how many different people she connected with through drumming and that she felt a sense of belonging to the group. Arisa loved the experience of being in the drum circle. She said the drum circle felt "so alive." She felt she was part of a living thing. Arisa discussed how while being inside the inner space of the drum circle she felt like she "was being cared for by the group." As a caregiver herself, Arisa recognized this action was a gift from the group and something which she longed for.

When the time came to paint a symbol of self onto the drum, Arisa reported that she did not think she could accomplish creating the image she imagined and that she wanted, because of her limited freehand painting skills. She created her own stencils of a Celtic knot circle in a quilting design to represent her Scottish heritage and lineage. She also created a dragon stencil. The dragon represented the wild animal inside that wanted to be free.

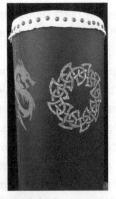 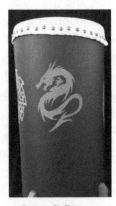 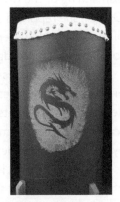

Figure A: Celtic knot circle   Figure B: Dragon   Figure C: Negative space dragon

Arisa immediately took the role of teacher and helped several members of the group create stencils and images of self on the drum. She was patient, kind and caring to members of the group. She demonstrated mastery in stencil making and painting despite her self-description of being a "crappy" painter.

Throughout the art and drumming experience, Arisa demonstrated various components of the ETC. She began with functioning on the Kinesthetic component through the physical act of drumming. Since she preferred to drum with her hands and specifically mentioned the tactile sensation of drumming, she appeared to find the Creative transition of the Kinesthetic/Sensory level of the ETC. She was able to entrain to the outside rhythm and expressed happiness from drumming indicating that she also found a balance on the Perceptual/Affective level of the ETC. Finally, Arisa used her engineering background to create stencils that represented her heritage, background and symbolic image of herself as a wild animal. This indicates functioning on the Cognitive/Symbolic level. Arisa demonstrated all levels of the ETC in a balanced manner suggesting that she was able to function on the Creative level of the ETC (Hinz 2009; Lusebrink 2010, 2016).

Arisa's mood improved during each drumming and art session. She expressed a more positive sense of self after the art and drumming experience. Throughout the drumming sessions, this facilitator provided unconditional positive regard, mirrored affect and modeled appropriate behavior within a safe and therapeutic space. Drum circle directives were employed to facilitate entrainment, group support and interactions while allowing for play (Hull 2006; Kossak 2015; Winnicott 2005). Arisa's style of attachment appeared to be secure through the activities of creating art and playing the drum within a therapeutic drum circle. These experiences of improvisational drumming and art making were novel experiences and Arisa appeared to thrive in terms of affect, attachment, sense of purpose and self-esteem.

Conclusion

This book describes the components required for creating a therapeutic drum circle that may prove to be beneficial to the participants' perceived sense of wellness (Mank 2019). The experience and results of the art and music making may prove to be beneficial, or therapeutic, to the participant even if the facilitator is not an art or music therapist and therefore is not practicing therapy. A drum circle is not considered music therapy unless a music therapist, within the context of a therapeutic alliance, facilitates the drum circle with the participants of the group. For this reason, the drum circles will be described as therapeutic drum circles and not music therapy. In order to attain entrainment and establish safety within a therapeutic drum circle, the facilitator should be familiar with the ETC in order to determine the functioning of the participants within the group and to devise an appropriate plan for drum circle directives with the goal of creative functioning (Hinz 2009; Hull 2006; Lusebrink 2010, 2016; Stevens 2017). A therapeutic space that allows for change is essential to therapeutic growth (Winnicott 2005), and change will be described in Chapter 2. Attachment styles, affect and purpose in life can change as a result of the therapeutic drum circle (Gillath *et al.* 2009; Mank 2019). The therapeutic drum circle provides a vehicle through which participants may achieve therapeutic growth and change while actively engaging in creativity (Hinz 2009; Lusebrink 1991, 2004, 2010, 2016; Mank 2019). This book provides the theories and instructions to build drums, make art, create music that holds potential to instill insight, and build attachment and healthy relationships while utilizing creativity.

CHAPTER 1

Art Therapy

Art therapy involves the making of art through any of the expressive mediums, including drawing, painting, photography or sculpture, as facilitated by an art therapist. The goal of art therapy is to improve the emotional, cognitive, physical and spiritual wellbeing of an individual (Rappaport 2009). The creative process of art making along with the therapeutic skills of an art therapist offer a means to address psychological and emotional issues that do not rely exclusively on verbal-based language (Moon 2008). Art therapy is often useful when traditional verbal-based therapies have proven to be unbeneficial to the client, as "art therapy engages the mind, body, and spirit in ways that are distinct from verbal articulation alone" (AATA 2020). The sensory-based nature of art making and art therapy engages the brain and the body in a manner that verbal language does not, offering alternative means to resolve issues, improve interpersonal skill sets, manage stress, and develop self-awareness and insight (AATA 2020). The process of achieving wellbeing through art therapy can take divergent paths, depending on the approach used by the art therapist.

Historical roots

Historically, the profession of art therapy provided two different constructs that offered paths to therapeutic healing, or wellbeing. The first approach, or construct, is known as "art as therapy" and incorporates the concept that the actual creation of art is "therapeutic and that the creative process is a growth-producing experience" (Malchiodi 2013). The second approach is "art psychotherapy" and holds that art is based in "symbolic communication" as a means to express feelings and an individual's personality (Malchiodi 2013). Both constructs can be used along a continuum to best serve the client depending on the specific and individualized goals of therapy (Malchiodi 2013). Employing creativity, through the arts, is considered to be inherently positive; it may lead to the enhancement of one's life and also promote healing (AATA 2020).

Despite the adherence to different art therapy constructs, art therapy is a profession, under the mental health discipline, where art therapists facilitate therapeutic interventions with the use of art mediums and the creative process to assist clients toward therapeutic growth and healing (AATA 2020). Art therapists are educated in psychological theories and art media practices in order to assist clients in employing artwork to uncover meaning. This discovery of meaning may benefit the client through addressing and improving emotional regulation, developing self-awareness, building self-esteem and social skills, and managing symptoms of mental illness (AATA 2020).

Art making offers an opportunity to express oneself and one's emotions, experiences, thoughts and reality through visual images or symbols. Through the use of color, line and shape an individual is offered the opportunity to convey meaning that words cannot. If an individual has "unresolved emotional experiences that occurred at the preverbal level, or possesses limited verbal capacity, art therapy provides a nonverbal means for conveying experience" (Rappaport 2009, p.69). The art acts as a language of its own, that is not dependent upon verbal language to communicate the inner reality of the artist, thereby offering opportunities for expression and healing through visual forms of expression (Rappaport 2009).

When utilizing art as therapy, the product takes a lesser role than that of the experience of creating the art (Malchiodi 2013). The experience of the making of the art and the emotions evoked in the maker are emphasized, while the art image or product is secondary to the art making experience. Dissanayake (1995) explains that all forms of art making and the art experience "facilitate a mood in which attention is focused, aroused, moved, manipulated, satisfied" (p.24). The essence of the art experience is that it is "physically pleasurable" (Dissanayake 1995, p.24).

Art and humans

In order to fully understand the value of art and art therapy, one must first look at the long relationship between humans, art and creativity. Art has played a role in most societies throughout history. There are examples of geometric patterns carved into ostrich egg shells found in Africa that date back hundreds of thousands of years (Cook & British Museum 2013). Anthropologists have found evidence of art and musical instruments originally constructed during the last Ice Age, which began 40,000 years ago and ended 12,000 years ago (Cook & British Museum 2013). Although it is well known that art existed in caves and in areas that were difficult to access, what may not be as universally known is that smaller and portable pieces existed and were displayed elsewhere in more accessible and commonly utilized spaces (Cook & British Museum 2013).

Small-sized art pieces and musical instruments were found among artifacts and the ruins of past societies. These items were once utilized in the tasks that comprised the typical daily routine of humans during the last Ice Age (Cook & British Museum 2013). In some cases, the portable art pieces were "specifically placed in pits or outside main areas of activities" and were "made with great skill of practiced artists" (Cook & British Museum 2013, p.12). This suggests that art and music were valued and utilized in the ordinary lives of modern humans and may have held a significant role within their culture and society. The use of art and music within the realms of the daily life of humans seems to attest to the human need for creativity, art and music, while affirming art as therapy (Dissanayake 1995; Malchiodi 2013).

Dissanayake (1995) states that the human desire, or drive, to create art is evident in all societies and cultures throughout the world. There is a sense of unity among people as a result of performing or witnessing an artistic event. There is often a sense of enjoyment, which is both physical and emotional, experienced by the individuals who are enjoined through the artistic experience (Dissanayake 1995).

This is an important concept to note when viewed within the context of survival. During the last Ice Age, for example, when the drive to stay warm, eat or reproduce would certainly be of utmost importance, humans took considerable time and effort to create art such as the Lion Person (Cook & British Museum 2013). The creator of this art object used their imagination to produce a sculpture that combined the features of a man with those of a lion. This sculpture took approximately 400 hours to complete, validating the theory that the act of creating art was a strong and powerful drive that held importance in previous cultures and societies (Cook & British Museum 2013).

Dissanayake (1995) expresses the idea that "what feels good is usually a cue to what we need" (p.32). The making of art and the prominent display in nearly every human society across time and the globe leads one to believe that art "fulfills a fundamental human need, satisfies an intrinsic and deep human imperative" (Dissanayake 1995, p.34). This need for creative expression is based in biology and is an innate and natural component of humans that connects them to nature and the natural environment. The behavior of creating and appreciating art throughout the evolution of man suggests that art was beneficial and helpful to the survival of humans who were involved in the creation or appreciation of art (Dissanayake 1995).

Humans have the ability to distinguish the ordinary from the extraordinary (Dissanayake 1995). By featuring and drawing attention to an object, behaviour or phenomenon through the creation of art, the ordinary is elevated to something distinctive and unusual. The object, behavior or phenomenon has been "made special" through the process of art making (Dissanayake 1995, p.42). It is within the environment of the making special process that exploration of the unknown can be evaluated, explored and understood. The making special process, which often contains a sense of play, can be controlled and protected so that understanding can take place (Dissanayake 1995). Others often witness the making special during certain events, celebrations or rituals. By incorporating the somatic senses in this way, the experience assumes greater importance and can become transformative, embodying something profound and a sense of potency that would not occur without the coming together of art and ritual. It is through the collaboration or ritual and making special that humans strive for the sublime or divine (Dissanayake 1995).

Art making with the art therapy process

Art also has the capacity to be a learning tool. Allen (1995) informs the reader that "[i]mages are a means of coming to know the richness and variety of our stories, their shadows and nuances" (p.10). Through the creation of art, an individual may structure or restructure their world to find meaning. Intention displayed in creating art requires the best efforts of the artist in order to achieve knowledge gained from the image and the unconscious (Allen 1995).

Allen (1995) emphasizes the value of the object being drawn or created. The selection of an item to be drawn or sculpted is important as it is a result of the powerful connection that exists between the artist and the object. The mindfulness of attending to the details of the object being created inspires focus, energy and ultimately a relationship between the artist and the object. The artist learns about the world and about the self as a result of the artistic process. The process of attending to the object brings awareness to the individual in regard to the individual's experience of emotions and self (Allen 1995).

Art therapy works to tap into the unconscious and guide the unconscious thoughts and feelings into conscious awareness (Rappaport 2009). Bringing thoughts and feelings into conscious awareness, through the creative process of art making, allows for an exploration of emotions and an evaluation of the perception of experiences. This process enables reflection upon one's own life and behaviour that may result in greater self-awareness and understanding of self. Art making and reflection on the information brought forth from the process allows for the possibility of change and offers an opportunity to learn new approaches and behaviors. It is through the process of art making and learning through creativity that one may find avenues out of negative and repetitive patterns of behavior (Allen 1995).

In the context of art therapy, art making is considered to contain the "intent to express some essential aspect of the human experience" (Moon 1998, p.8). The art therapist attends to the client under the aegis of the image making process by being present, making art with the client and acting in a manner that honors the existence of the client and the artwork created (Moon 1998). The witnessing of the artwork is paramount in the therapeutic environment as it allows for a reflection on the process and the information offered by way of the image itself. The act of witnessing the art created is a means to provide respect for the artwork, the process and the image. In doing so, one must adopt a nonjudgmental mindset that is one of acceptance of what is offered through the art therapy process (Moon 1998). Moon (1998, 2008) describes the art therapy process as being meta-verbal or beyond words. Therefore, verbal communication is not often necessary, as an understanding may become known simply through the act of creating and witnessing the art within the therapeutic environment.[1]

The practice of art therapy is dependent on a host of variables, including the length and setting of treatment, the goals and needs of the client and those of the society in which the client resides, culture, theoretical orientation of the therapist, and the experiences of both the client and the therapist (Bucciarelli 2016). The art created within an art therapy relationship is reflective of the client's reality, which is influenced and shaped by the experience of the society in which the client resides (Allen 1995). The political climate, social values and cultural practices all coalesce to form a sense of reality for an individual, which becomes the tenor within the art created during an art therapy session (Allen 1995). The process of honoring, touching or caressing the art has the power to build rapport and attunement within the therapeutic relationship (Hass-Cohen, Kim & Mangassarian 2015).

The art therapist's role is to attend to the client as well as to the art. It is essential to the therapeutic relationship that the art therapist is capable of being present in the therapeutic moment, is willing to create with the client and is ardent in supporting and expressing value toward the client and the artwork (Allen 1995). Naumburg (1973) and Ulman (2001) hypothesized that art, within the therapeutic experience, is the mechanism of change. The art must be honored, accepted and allowed to express the thoughts, needs and emotions of the client.

Neuroscience and art therapy

While the art itself is of great significance, the activity and processing occurring within the brain and the body's reaction to making and viewing art cannot be overlooked. Until recently, art therapists showed a reluctance to align with science and preferred to favor an art-focused philosophy and approach to the practice of art therapy (Malchiodi 2012). Scientific findings concerning "how images influence emotion, thoughts and well-being" are changing the strict art-focused approach (Malchiodi 2012, p.16). The scientific findings indicate a mind and

---

1   Allen (1995) discusses "knowing" and the process of knowing things. Understanding is a result of intention, witnessing and reflection. In this case understanding does not occur but rather is a process of knowing.

body connection that is impacted by the experience of creating art (Malchiodi 2012). The mind and body theory posits that the mind has a significant effect on the health of the body (Malchiodi 2012).

According to Malchiodi (2012), through neuroscience, or the study of the brain and its capabilities, data is emerging that suggests that the "brain, human physiology, and emotions are intricately intertwined" (p.17). The knowledge base concerning early attachment and its impact on neurological processes throughout the lifespan of the individual, along with the effects of trauma on cognitive processing and memory of the individual, has increased as a result of the neurologically based research founded in art therapy intervention (Chapman 2014; Chapman *et al.* 2001; Malchiodi 2012). Malchiodi (2012) writes that "science will be central to the understanding and defining how art therapy actually works and why it is a powerful therapeutic modality" (p.17).

Belkofer and Konopka (2008) conducted a single-subject research study that employed electroencephalography (EEG) to measure brain activity in an individual at rest and then after one hour of drawing and painting. The EEG measures brain wave frequencies and amplitude through the electrodes in a headpiece attached to the head of the individual being studied. The resulting data from the EEG single-subject study indicated that there was a significant difference ($p < .05$) in brain activity after one hour of art making (Belkofer & Konopka 2008) Two regions associated with increased brain wave activity were the occipital and parietal lobes, which are associated with visual-spatial and perceptual processing (Belkofer & Konopka 2008). The temporal lobe is the area of the brain involved with processing image meaning, memory and spirituality, and was also recorded by the EEG as having increased activity (Belkofer & Konopka 2008). The limbic system is located within the temporal lobe and is associated with the formation of emotions (Belkofer & Konopka 2008).

The significance of the temporal lobe activity suggests that memories associated with emotional states may be activated through art making (Belkofer & Konopka 2008). This study provided information that located specific brain structures which were influenced by creating and viewing art. The brain controls all processes of the body; therefore, when the brain is activated, the body is influenced and when the body is activated, the brain is influenced (Malchiodi 2012). The EEG data from the Belkofer and Konopka (2008) study suggests that the mind–body connection is stimulated as a result of art creation and viewing, giving credence to the art therapy theories that art making is the mechanism of change within the art therapy relationship.

Expressive Therapies Continuum

Positron emission tomography (PET) and magnetic resonance imaging (MRI) provide evidence that supports the theories of a connection between visual imagery and artistic expression and the brain (King 2016; Lusebrink 2004). These tests also validate the theory that both hemispheres of the brain are activated as a result of art images (King 2016). The act of creating art evokes fundamental changes within the body, emotions and the structural level of the brain (King 2016; Lusebrink 2004, 2010, 2016). The ability of the brain to change and form new connections throughout an individual's life is known as neuroplasticity (King 2016).

Lusebrink (2004) discusses the functions of several of the known brain structures that may be impacted by the expressive arts. The structures of the brain have specific functions and vary in the complexity of processing. King (2016) and Lusebrink (2004) add that the cognitive processing within these structures is conducted consciously as well as unconsciously. The brain structures also offer alternative pathways for "accessing and processing visual and motor information and memories" (Lusebrink 2004) should there be a need, as a result of physical or psychiatric reasons. Art therapy has the capacity to utilize the alternative pathways, or neuroplasticity, of the brain (Hinz 2009; King 2016; Lusebrink 2004, 2016). Art therapy offers continued and alternative opportunities for the brain to continue to process stimuli in the event of a blockage that inhibits processing in the primary pathway or brain structure, as a result of trauma and/or physiological or emotional issues (Hinz 2009; King 2016, Lusebrink 2004, 2016). The vast array of art materials and art media offer opportunities for the art therapist to identify possible blockages within the "processing of information and emotions" and work to improve the integration of emotional and cognitive information by way of the art therapy process (Lusebrink 2004).

Lusebrink (2010) identifies criteria that differentiate art therapy from verbal-based therapy. Art therapy offers an opportunity to express emotions and foster communication through the creation of art. The artwork provides a mechanism to express emotions on either a nonverbal or verbal level. The image itself conveys "multileveled meaning present in visual expression and the therapeutic effects of the creative process" (Lusebrink 2010). Emotions, experience or knowledge are revealed through the visual medium as a result of the processing of the information via the visual information processing system within the occipital and temporal lobes of the brain (Lusebrink 2010). The art image contains emotional content and offers the opportunity to express, process and inform the creator (Lusebrink 2004, 2010). The ETC provides a schematic, or theoretical, framework that delineates the cognitive processes which emanate within specific brain regions and structures as a result of the art therapy experience (Hinz 2009; Lusebrink 2004, 2010, 2016).

The ETC is a theoretical framework that provides a visual representation of how an individual processes information and stimuli (Hinz 2009; Lusebrink 2004, 2016). It is a model comprising three hierarchical bipolar levels along with the Creative level (Hinz 2009; Lusebrink 2004, 2016). Each pole of a level represents possible pathology that may be represented within the visual images created (Hinz 2009; Lusebrink 2004, 2010, 2016). It is possible for an individual to linearly progress laterally and vertically across and between levels of the ETC. The bipolar levels comprise a hierarchical structure that ranges from simple to complex (Lusebrink 2016). The three bipolar levels are Kinesthetic/Sensory, Perceptual/Affective, Cognitive/Symbolic. These levels depict a progression of cognitive development and processing that is reflective within the art image and in the media selected to create it. The Creative transition represents a central point between the two poles within a level that is a balance of both aspects of that level. The Creative level does not have separate poles and is the balance and integration of all of the levels. The Creative level offers potential for an individual to function in a cohesive and creative manner (Hinz 2009; Lusebrink 2004, 2010, 2016).

Kinesthetic/Sensory level

The level of the ETC that is considered the least complex is the Kinesthetic/Sensory level. It is represented by simple motor movement that is focused upon the discharge of physical energy of the art making process necessary to create visual imagery through a variety of art mediums and forms (Hinz 2009). The Kinesthetic component is characterized by a diverse range of energy that is expressed through increased, or intense, energy or through an insufficient level of arousal or energy necessary to complete the task of art making (Lusebrink 2016). If the individual's attention is focused toward the Kinesthetic component, then the art expression can be identified through intense movements without the conscious awareness of boundaries, or by an insufficient level of arousal or energy level that is necessary to complete the art expression (Lusebrink 2016). Within the painting of a drum, the Kinesthetic component functioning within a participant could be demonstrated by the splashing of paint or through the dropping of brushes loaded with paint onto the surface of the drum wall. The inability to move the paintbrush could also depict functioning in the Kinesthetic component. Lusebrink (2016) theorized that the basal ganglia and primary motor cortex within the brain are activated during the kinesthetic processing of expressive art making (Lusebrink 2016).

If the Sensory component, or pole, is activated during art making within the expressive arts, then the focus is based upon the tactile or visual aspects of the art materials selected and used in the art making process (Hinz 2009; Lusebrink 1991; 2010, 2016). The characteristics of the Sensory pole include recognition of, and sensitivity to, sensory stimuli with slow, or controlled or measured, movements. Within the context of painting a symbol of self upon the drum, the sensory component could be demonstrated through slow brush strokes while the participant focused upon the colors of the paint or the tactile sensations of the paint on the tube, or visually connected to the painting process and color painted on the drum. The primary somato-sensory cortex of the brain is theorized to be activated and stimulated at this pole. A balance at the Kinesthetic/ Sensory level, or the Creative transition within this level, is exemplified by a kinesthetic and sensory awareness of the artistic materials and movements resulting from the art making experience (Hinz 2009; Lusebrink 2010, 2016).

As a result of the creative process, there is an opportunity for increased and more complex levels of functioning to emerge, defined as the emergent function of each level of the ETC (Hinz 2009; Lusebrink 1991). The emergent function is the expression of a variety of characteristics, including attributes from the subsequent, or higher, level within the ETC. The emergent function of the Kinesthetic pole is characterized by an increase in form and boundaries. The emergent function of the Sensory pole involves an emphasis upon emotions, or the affective experience of the art making process (Hinz 2009).

The reflective distance is defined as the time difference between a stimulus and the reaction to that specific stimulus (Hinz 2009; Lusebrink 1991). The response time involves necessary amount of time it takes for the individual to cognitively process the art making experience (Hinz 2009). There is a positive relationship between the reflective distance and the complexity of the hierarchical levels of the ETC, meaning that as the hierarchical levels increase there is a greater time differential in the reaction to the stimulus by the individual (Lusebrink 1991).

In short, the Kinesthetic/Sensory level is defined as the simplest and most fundamental level of the ETC in regard to the intricacy of development and processing of emotions and cognitions (Lusebrink 1991). The Kinesthetic/Sensory level has a short reflective distance exemplified by the length of time between the stimulus of movement and the subsequent reaction, or emotional response, to the gross motor movement associated with the art medium selected and expressed. The reflective distance at the Kinesthetic/Sensory level is considered to be low. The reflective distance is the product of the spontaneous attributes of the art expression, the enterprise of creation, the personal experience of the actual art form, and the corporeal and subsequent emotional response to the art experience (Lusebrink 1991). Within the realm of drumming, individuals are often fully engrossed in rhythm, movement and sound, resulting in a reduction of capability for cognitive reflection or processing. As the drum is struck or played, and sound is then produced, there is opportunity for movement across the Kinesthetic/Sensory level towards the Sensory pole. Therefore, drumming may be viewed as a representation of the sensorimotor phase of human development—that is, the comprehensive inclusion of sound and gross motor movement (Lusebrink 1991).

Perceptual/Affective level

The next, and more complex, level within the hierarchical model of the ETC is the Perceptual/Affective level. The emphasis within this level is upon forms, boundaries and emotional experiences. The Perceptual pole of this level is focused upon form and boundaries, whereas the Affective pole is associated with the expression of emotions. The Perceptual pole is distinguished by clear, defined areas and boundaries, or by a lack, or dissolution, of boundaries and fragmentation of forms. The symbol of self that is painted on the drum could offer opportunities to paint in abstract forms that are defined or that blend into the contrasting shapes and colors painted on the drum. The symbol could be completely defined or be partial elements of form and structure. The emphasis at the Perceptual pole is upon formal art elements, including form, line, color and a differentiation of figure and ground. It is theorized that the ventral stream of the inferior temporal lobe is stimulated when an individual is processing on the Perceptual pole (Lusebrink 2016).

The expression of emotion, or affect, is representative of functioning at the Affective pole (Hinz 2009; Lusebrink 2010, 2016). Affective pole functioning is identified by intensification of value and hue within the artwork. Each pole has divergent or opposite characteristics that are indicative of functioning at the particular pole. Affective pole functioning may also include the use of inappropriate color to represent the subject matter of the image, or the symbol on the drum, and may also be depicted by the lack of discrimination between figure and ground (Lusebrink 2016). The amygdala within the brain is stimulated and activated when an individual is functioning at the Affective pole as emotions are processed during, and as a result of, the art making experience (Lusebrink 2016). The Creative transition region of the Perceptual/Affective level is exemplified by the configuration of rich, colorful and artistic forms, as well as by the processing of positive gestalts (Lusebrink 2016). The emergent function of the Perceptual pole is composed of an increase in cognitive processing and self-awareness, along with an increased ability to verbally express, evaluate and categorize experiences (Hinz 2009). The emergent function of the Affective pole includes the ability to identify and embody emotions, determine the meaning of symbolic images, and associate personal significance within the artwork and art making experience (Hinz 2009).

Cognitive/Symbolic level

The most complex visual information processing occurs at the Cognitive/Symbolic level of the ETC (Hinz 2009). The Cognitive pole is associated with stimulation of the prefrontal cortex of the brain; the emphasis of the Symbolic pole is based in the processing of personal and often private information as well as its expression in symbolic form. The Symbolic pole stimulates the orbitofrontal cortex and the cingulate cortex of the brain (Lusebrink 2016). At the Cognitive/Symbolic level, the emphasis is focused upon cognitive processing and how the gestalts comprising lines and shapes climax in concept development, conscious comprehension of spatial components, and verbal expression within the art and expressive arts representation (Lusebrink 2016). The art expression often evokes deep emotional content, especially when creating a symbol of self on the drum. The contrasting aspect of the Cognitive pole is represented as the reversal of figure and ground and in the form of peculiar symbols (Lusebrink 2016). The Creative transition area is portrayed by images or art expressions that induce spirituality, intuition and a greater understanding of self (Lusebrink 2016). The emergent function of the Cognitive pole is the ability to utilize creative approaches that incorporate verbalization, imagination and symbolism in order to find solutions to specific problems. The emergent function of the Symbolic pole is the increased ability to identify unique, and previously unknown, aspects of self. The discovery of new aspects of self allows for the acquisition of inner wisdom that is incorporated and integrated into the self, allowing for an increase in self-esteem, which provides opportunity for advances in personal freedom (Hinz 2009).

Art processing and the Expressive Therapies Continuum

Conceptualizing the art making processes via the theoretical framework of the ETC provides an opportunity for the art therapist to identify client strengths and blockages during the cognitive processing of information along and between the levels within the ETC (Hinz 2009; Lusebrink 2004, 2010, 2016). Art therapy practices and specific art mediums can be effectively employed to facilitate integrative functioning within levels while working to achieve Creative transitions between the poles on each level. As the client progresses in effectively processing information, the integration between levels can provide Creative level processing and functioning. The strengths and weaknesses of the individual are assessed, identified and ultimately addressed to aid the individual in reducing problematic and pathological behavior. The initiation point within the

ETC framework is the level or component that is most comfortable for the individual (Lusebrink 2016). The subsequent movement from the initiation point to higher levels within the ETC framework is gradual, with the intention to reduce the probability of overwhelming the client (Hinz 2009).

The four levels of the ETC encompass a progression of information processing by the individual that is illustrated in the graphic representations from Kinesthetic/Sensory to Perceptual/Affective and Cognitive/Symbolic (Hinz 2009). As a client works with an art therapist in a therapeutic alliance, the art therapist is guided by the ETC theoretical framework in assessing the client's visual and cognitive processing through art and the utilization of a variety of art mediums. An individual has the opportunity to traverse laterally or vertically through the spectrum of levels of the ETC accessing the varied healing properties of art therapy while utilizing art mediums that correspond to the four levels of the ETC (Hinz 2009). The ETC is a comprehensive, theoretical framework that provides opportunities to enlist a variety of art mediums to obtain a descriptive inventory of a client's strengths and challenges. The ETC provides a visual portrayal of the diverse levels of cognitive processing and functioning within the brain of the individual (Hinz 2009; Lusebrink 2004, 2010, 2016).

Brain structures and the ETC

Ogden, Pain and Fisher (2006) deliberate the theory that the brain comprises hierarchical systems that have evolved as a response to the need for processing and responding to exposure to diverse stimuli. The first level to develop within the human brain was the "reptilian brain (comprised of the brain stem and cerebellum) which govern arousal, homeostasis of the organism, reproductive drives, sensation and instinctual movement impulses, the heart of sensorimotor experience" (p.5).

The next brain structure to develop was the paleomammalian brain, which is also known as the limbic brain. The limbic system is a universal structure found in every mammal. Its purpose is to regulate and oversee the physical and emotional experiences, memory, social behavior, and knowledge acquisition of an individual (Ogden *et al.* 2006).

The neocortex was the last brain structure to develop within the brain in the evolution of humans. The neocortex oversees cognitive and executive functioning, self awareness, and identification and conceptual recognition (Ogden *et al.* 2006). This hierarchical theory purports that all three systems are necessary to enable human beings to think abstractly, possess self-awareness, express emotions, and process disparate stimuli (Ogden *et al.* 2006).

The hierarchical system is reliant upon the adequate functioning of the cognitive, emotional and sensorimotor levels in order to effectively and efficiently process stimuli and experiential information (Ogden *et al.* 2006). The highest level of processing capability is the Cognitive level that integrates the information provided by the lower level brain structures composed of the limbic and reptilian brain structures. Effective processing within the Cognitive level requires integration of the lower levels in order to provide accurate information based on the sensorimotor and the somatosensory systems (Ogden *et al.* 2006). The "top down" approach refers to an integrated hierarchical system that has the capacity for cognitively processing information in order to organize plans and provide structure for the purpose of accomplishing preselected and specified goals (Ogden *et al.* 2006, p.4). A "bottom up" approach of the hierarchical system relies on information provided by body sensations and instinct to direct and inform cognitive processing and functioning (Ogden *et al.* 2006).

Dysregulation of the autonomic system, often a result of trauma, can result in the loss of cognitive processing (or "top down" processing) and is often represented by behavior based entirely upon sensorimotor and emotional experience or by a "bottom up" approach (Ogden *et al.* 2006). Through the ETC, a visual representation of the type of brain processing and potential blockages can be observed in the art image and art making process (Hinz 2009; Lusebrink 2016). The art therapist is able to utilize art-based, experiential directives to facilitate an individual's cognitive processing abilities along the ETC to evolve to a more cohesive and integrated form (Hinz 2009; Lusebrink 2016).

The ETC has the capacity to address the needs of the individual by providing a means by which the art therapist may assess and identify the specific brain systems the client utilizes most frequently. A linear approach, within the ETC, is incorporated by the art therapist to stimulate and integrate other structures of the brain in order to reduce or eliminate pathological behavior and thereby increase creativity

(Hinz 2009). The ETC framework and hierarchy guides the art therapist in activating and navigating between processing systems in a person-centered approach that addresses the specific needs of each individual. The levels within the ETC provide information on the cognitive and emotional processing of information, allowing for expression of an individual's personal experience via the artistic process (Lusebrink 2016).

The theoretical framework of the ETC guides and informs the therapist and the art therapy directives employed to assist in identifying blockages that are occurring within or between levels of the ETC in the brain structures of the client (Hinz 2009). Art therapy and art mediums, which relate to specific levels of the ETC, may be implemented with the goal of integrating functioning associated with the hierarchical levels within the brain and the ETC (Hinz 2009; Lusebrink 2016). This process works to facilitate Creative transitions between the various poles within each level (Luzebrink 2016). The ETC, in conjunction with art therapy, provides a means to identify, assess and address the individual's strengths and weaknesses. The initiation point of art therapy lies in the art medium that the client is most comfortable using and is indicative a specific level of the theoretical framework of the ETC (Lusebrink 2016). Hinz (2009) advises traversing from the initiation point in a gradual, linear process to reduce the possibility of overwhelming the client or individual (Hinz 2009).

Neuroplasticity

Hass-Cohen and Findlay (2015) introduce the Art Therapy Relational Neuroscience (ATR-N) as a means to assist art therapists in selecting and implementing specific neurobiological art interventions that will best meet the specific needs of the client. Hass-Cohen and Findlay (2015) assert that art therapy is a means to express emotions and that through this process therapeutic change and healing can begin. Art making, within the art therapy process, stimulates specific areas of the brain and may activate the process of neuroplasticity through the building of new neurons and connections (Hass-Cohen & Findlay 2015). The ATR-N consists of six principles represented in the acronym CREATE: Creative embodiment, Relational resonating, Expressive communicating, Adaptive responding, Transformative integrating and Empathizing and compassion (Hass-Cohen & Findlay 2015). The principles seek to capture the powerful and evolving nature of the brain and its ability to adapt and transform in response to stimuli and physical or mental activity (Hass-Cohen & Findlay 2015).

Hass-Cohen and Findlay (2015) employ visual imagery through the art mediums of sculpture, drawing and painting to activate the visual process within individuals. Vision and visual processing are essential to human survival and provide an individual with a synthesized view of the world. Hass-Cohen and Findlay (2015) utilize art experientials, based in the varied art mediums, to gain a new understanding of the world that spans from the abstract to the kinetic.

Storytelling and written responses to the art created can act as vital components of the therapeutic process. Often responses to the artwork are written and used as a method of moving from the preverbal to the verbal method of communication within the art therapy process (Block, Harris & Laing 2005). Written art reflection activates the cognitive functions, emotion regulation and social interaction areas of the higher regions of the brain and encourages learning by way of creativity (Hass-Cohen & Findlay 2015).

Successful and effective therapeutic change requires experiential modalities that incorporate emotional and intellectual components to convert experience into knowledge (Hass-Cohen & Findlay 2015). The multi-modal approach incorporates imagination and psychological and neurobiological theory along with sensory and aesthetic experiences to stimulate neuroplasticity and effect long-term therapeutic change and healing (Hass-Cohen & Findlay 2015). ATR-N and CREATE offer a mind–body approach to healing through the art making and reflection process based in neurobiology and art therapy.

Social interactions with people and one's environment form the basis of relational neuroscience and utilize attachment theory (Hass-Cohen & Findlay 2015). Social interactions mold and change the wiring of the brain throughout the lifespan of an individual. The type and quality of social interactions enhance or decrease the coping mechanisms of the individual (Hass-Cohen & Findlay 2015). Neural growth within the hippocampus of the brain, brain development and reorganization, along with positive interactions and experiences may be causal factors in the formation of resiliency (Hass-Cohen & Findlay 2015). Resiliency is the integration and effective response to daily life stressors and negative experience that may lead to a higher quality of life (Richardson 2002).

It is important to note that art therapy facilitates a mind–body connection through the manipulation of art materials, along with positive relationship building between the client and the therapist and cognitive reflection on the artwork (Hass-Cohen & Findlay 2015). The therapeutic relationship and milieu contribute to mindfulness and this is the basis of compassion and empathy for oneself and others (Hass-Cohen & Findlay 2015). Utilizing the CREATE and ATR-N model for therapeutic change may result in better coping skills, compassion and neuroplasticity in the individual.

Broderick (2011) confirms that "art therapies are therapeutic interventions informed by the practice of psychology, psychotherapy and psychiatry" (p.96). The therapeutic relationship and the interventions employed by the art therapist differentiate between art making and art therapy. Art is based in creations while art therapy is founded in service and healing (Broderick 2011). Within the art therapy process, art making is used as a "tool for recovery" (Broderick 2011).

Conclusion

Art therapy provides the tools for expression, healing and resilience (AATA 2020). Studies indicate that the brain changes as a result of the kinesthetic movement that occurs within art making and mindfulness practice, and as a result of the visual processes needed for the creation of the art (Hass-Cohen & Findlay 2015; Hinz 2009; Lusebrink 2004). The therapeutic relationship between the art therapist and the client offers social communication, relationship building and modeling, as well as a platform for understanding through the arts (Hass-Cohen & Findlay 2015; Hinz 2009). Art therapy offers the opportunity for discovery and change, no matter whether it is viewed as art as therapy or art psychotherapy. The process of creating art in a mindful manner that includes thoughtful witnessing and processing of the art has the potential to lead to therapeutic change and to provide knowledge and understanding that may lead to greater self-awareness (Allen 1995; Hass-Cohen & Findlay 2015).

CHAPTER 2

Psychodynamic Theory

Freud

Psychodynamic theory originated with Freud's theories on human behavior and subsequent techniques in counseling categorized as psychoanalysis (Koffmann & Walters 2014). Freud was interested in the personal, or subjective, experience of the individual that drove their actions and behavior throughout life. The childhood experience of each individual forms the template that governs and propels them to develop their own idiosyncratic perspective of the world (Koffmann & Walters 2014).

Freud strove to eliminate psychological and emotional suffering in individuals through the process of psychoanalysis and psychodynamic theory (Bienenfeld 2005). Freud's theories of psychoanalysis are based on two premises: psychodeterminism and the dynamic unconscious. Psychodeterminism is the presumption that an individual's mental processing and activity is not random, but rather is connected to, and a result of, preceding thoughts and experiences. The psychoeducation provided by the therapist could influence therapeutic change, albeit briefly, within the individual seeking therapeutic assistance. Bienenfeld (2005) states that "[w]ith enough effort and creativity, it is possible to assign meaning to all of our thoughts, feelings, behavior, dreams and mistakes" (p.7).

The dynamic unconscious premise posits that the majority of mental processing of an individual occurs outside of conscious perception (Bienenfeld 2005). Therefore, psychodeterminism is reliant upon a dynamic unconsciousness that is actively working to process information and motivations. The connection of thoughts and ideas is often hidden within the unconscious mental processing of an individual (Bienenfeld 2005).

Levels of consciousness

Freud theorized that there exists a "system of awareness" within the mind of each individual (Bienenfeld 2005, p.8). The system comprises three levels of consciousness, each consisting of a tumult of mental activity. The three levels are termed as conscious, preconscious and unconscious (Bienenfeld 2005; Rubin 2001). Each level of mental activity influences and compels the behavior of an individual (Bienenfeld 2005; Rubin 2016). The conscious level consists of mental processing that is within the awareness of the individual and is readily accessible through the thoughts "on one's mind" (Rubin 2001, p.16). The mental processing within the preconscious level is not yet in the awareness of the individual, although it is available to the individual (Bienenfeld 2005; Rubin 2001). The mental processing at the unconscious level is "concealed by the conscious awareness" and is capable of revealing itself through "indirect manifestations" of behavior on the part of the individual (Bienenfeld 2005, p.9).

The energy that stimulates and arouses an individual is defined as a drive (Bienenfeld 2005). There exist two types of drive, which are biologically based impulses entailing either an aggressive or sexual compulsion (Bienenfeld 2005). The sexual drive stimulates the individual toward "reproduction, connection and affection" (Bienenfeld 2005, p.8). The aggressive drive spurs the individual toward disruption and disintegration of social connections. Drives are not within the conscious awareness of the individual, and they create anxiety or excitement as a result of fulfillment or reconciliation of the impulse (Bienenfeld 2005).

Tripartite division of the mind

Freud expanded upon the ideas of drives and systems of awareness to include a "tripartite division of the mind" (Rubin 2001, p.16). The tripartite division encompasses the Id, Ego and Superego and exists outside of conscious awareness (Bienenfeld 2005; Rubin 2001, 2016). The Id is the first of the mental structures to develop, is founded in both sexual and aggressive drives, and is nonverbal (Bienenfeld 2005; Rubin 2001). The Id has no quantifiable sense of time as it developed prior to a sense of self and autonomy (Bienenfeld 2005). The forbidden urges of the drives within the Id are often repressed desires and they strive for fulfillment through covert means in order to elude the censorship of the Ego (Rubin 2001, 2016). The true nature of the desire and the observable behavior is not accessible to conscious awareness.

The Ego is responsible for satisfying the urges from the drives of the Id (Bienenfeld 2005; Rubin 2001, 2016). The Ego is capable of motor functions that include physical movement of the body, and its cognitive abilities entail memory allowing for "delayed gratification of id impulses" if needed (Bienenfeld 2005, p.10). The process of satisfying the impulses from the Id can be accomplished through straightforward, rechanneled or temporized means (Bienenfeld 2005).

The Super Ego mental structure holds the cultural and moral standards of the individual (Bienenfeld 2005; Rubin 2001). The Super Ego and the Ego regulate how, if and when the impulses from the Id will be expressed (Bienenfeld 2005; Rubin 2001). The standards of the Ego are also evaluated and possibly incorporated during this process of examination.

Freud theorized that thoughts, dream content and Id impulses that are repressed are termed latent (Bienenfeld 2005; Rubin 2001). Freud's theories and techniques strove to move latent and repressed traumatic memories from the unconscious to the conscious awareness with the goal of insight, awareness and therapeutic healing (Rubin 2001). Catharsis, or the moving of the repressed thoughts and memories from unconscious to conscious awareness, was believed to be the pivotal means to achieve therapeutic recovery and healing (Rubin 2001).

Psychodynamic theory and art therapy

Freud also identified the fact that individuals convey dreams and memories verbally in terms of visual imagery (Rubin 2001). Naumburg, one of the first people documented to use art as a therapeutic tool, recognized the importance of making art to express dreams and fantasies in order to achieve catharsis within the therapeutic relationship (Naumburg 1973; Rubin 2001). Naumberg looked at the creation of art as the primary tool in moving the unconscious to the conscious level of mental processing, and termed her method "dynamically oriented art therapy" (Rubin 2001, p.17).

Naumburg viewed "the patient's artwork as symbolic speech," thereby acknowledging the creator of the artwork as the primary owner of knowledge in the symbolic meaning of the artwork (Rubin 2001, p.17). Another therapeutic intervention within psychodynamic theory is free association. Naumburg (1973) used free association in conjunction with the art created to uncover latent and often emotionally charged meaning contained within the art. Through the facilitation of the therapeutic process, the art therapist guides and supports the client while the client discovers the symbolic meaning of the image.

The meaning making through the art therapy process is another form of making special. Making special by way of making art, or aesthetic making special, propels the individual from an emotional state, presumably without anxiety, to a state of change, which is anxiety provoking, and then into a new and integrated state that is devoid of anxiety (Dissanayake 1995). These changes are often highly charged and hold great significance to the individuals involved (Dissanayake 1995). Moving from a neutral emotional state into a state of anxiety and then beyond often evokes a sense of boundary dissolution and a timeless connection to something more or greater than the individual and is known as the liminal phase (Dissanayake 1995).

The liminal phase, or transitional phase, is frequently discussed within the realm of art therapy. Art and the aesthetic experience are central components leading to therapeutic change through the use of art therapy. Naumburg (1973) emphasizes that art, within the context of art therapy, is used to "explore and reintegrate human personality" (p.49). Naumberg used extemporaneous art making to expose the unconscious and believed that this was a cathartic and curative experience that employed imagery to communicate repressed impulses (Naumburg 1973; Rubin 2001; Ulman 2001).

Transference and countertransference

Art making combined with the Freudian principles of transference and countertransference were the primary methods Naumberg (1973) utilized as a means to offer therapeutic help to children diagnosed with a mental illness. Transference occurs when the client unconsciously attributes characteristics onto the therapist that are nonexistent or are not as amplified as the client perceives (Gilroy & McNeilly 2000). Transference is a powerful therapeutic tool that can be employed to explore past experiences and perceptions. The purpose is to explore other possible meanings of the experience or the perception that may result in a positive outcome and therapeutic growth for the client (Gilroy & McNeilly 2000).

Schaverien (1999) characterizes transference between a client and a verbal-based therapist as the client unconsciously projecting the client's inner perceptions of the world onto the therapist. The role of the therapist is to work with the client to find alternatives to the inner conflict and discover a resolution to past issues or problems. When working with an art therapist while utilizing art psychotherapy, the art acts to form a triad between the client, the therapist and the image (Schaverien 1999). The image embodies the role of the container for the emotions expressed, thereby allowing the client to objectively evaluate the situation while witnessing the symbolism expressed from the unconscious. Schaverien (1992) theorizes that countertransference occurs when the art therapist expresses approval, appreciation and acceptance of the artwork created by the client. The appreciation of the image works to illuminate and validate the acceptance of the client who created the art and positively builds upon the growing therapeutic relationship (Schaverien 1992).

Both verbal-based therapy and art therapy use transference and countertransference to facilitate therapeutic healing; however, the process is different. By projecting the transference onto an image, the client has the opportunity to experience the artwork with a detached demeanor. It is through the appreciation of the artwork created while holding an objective stance, thereby neutralizing distressing emotions, that the client is able to obtain an aesthetic experience (Dissanayake 1995). De Botton & Armstrong (2013) state that "[a]rt can offer a grand and serious vantage point from which to survey the travails of our condition" (p.30). It is through the aesthetic experience that a client is able to utilize transference to gain perspective and insight and to work toward therapeutic growth.

Naumburg (1973) utilized the process of psychodynamic therapy in conjunction with art creation to assist clients in accessing parts of the client's personality. This was accomplished by using the symbolic language of art to reach the unconscious, thereby releasing inner wishes, fears, desires and inner conflicts. Via the free expression of art, or the authentic experience, an individual has the opportunity to expose difficulties within, reveal past traumatic experience and create opportunities that have potential to lead to an understanding of the situation or aberrant behavior; ultimately this may result in therapeutic healing. The authentic experience of creative expression is in essence a language for communication while becoming a source for therapeutic healing and growth regardless of one's mental health (Naumburg 1973).

Sublimation and art therapy

Another concept pioneered by Freud is sublimation, and it is categorized as a technique within psychodynamic theory. Edith Kramer worked with children, employing art therapy, to substantiate and improve upon the theory of sublimation while incorporating symbolism (Rubin 1987). Kramer (1972) characterizes sublimation as the "process in which a primitive asocial impulse is transformed into a socially productive act" (p.41). Sublimation acts to redirect the instinctual drives and energy of the Id, by way of the Ego, producing socially acceptable forms through the use of art making (Kramer 2001). Sublimation is a multi-step, ego-syntonic process that involves an object holding interest, a designated goal and energy to redirect the impulse to a new, different and more socially acceptable goal that supports and strengthens the ego (Kramer 2001). Imagination takes precedence over fantasy, allowing symbolism to be evoked and acted upon through the artistic process of art making within the therapeutic tool of sublimation (Kramer 2001).

The positive emotions felt from the socially acceptable act are a replacement for the emotional release that the asocial act would have provided. The use of art making, as a method of sublimation, acts to transform the primal impulse through the creation of an abstract structure that consists of symbolic language free from anxiety (Kramer 1972, 2001). The process of sublimation and art making reduces the urge for the individual to display impulsive, asocial behavior (Kramer 1972, 2001).

Kramer (2001) provided a therapeutic environment in which to work with children. Within the therapeutic environment of the open studio, Kramer assisted children in the creation of art pieces that symbolized the pain and suffering the child was experiencing, with the goal of achieving catharsis within the child. Kramer (2001) served as the support the child required in order to traverse through the emotionally charged impulses in an attempt to gain insight. Art therapists help direct the client to modify behavior or choose materials that will effectively evoke expression in a controlled and manageable manner (Kramer 2001). The art therapist may provide materials and interventions, including tearing paper, shaping clay, or a medium that appropriately matches the emotions currently experienced by the client. The art therapist may actively use positive reframing to discuss and describe the actions or behavior of the client. Positive reframing is a technique employed by the art therapist to re-direct attention, thereby allowing the individual to focus upon modifying behavior and affect. The actions of the therapist create a situation that allows for the expression and release of the impulses being experienced without added distress to the client (Kramer 2001). The therapist is integral to the sublimation process—their support is required as the client may not possess sufficient skills to effectively cause redirection of the impulses from the Id in order to meet societal standards of acceptable behavior (Kramer 2001).

Sublimation and drumming

The making of a drum has the potential to incorporate the concepts of sublimation by way of transforming an individual's primitive impulses through the symbolic language of art that is created upon the drum. Asocial impulses could be redirected into art making or through the kinesthetic movements of drumming. The art materials selected have the potential to match and redirect the energy of the asocial impulses toward the aesthetic experience (Dissanayake 1995; Kramer 2001; Robbins 1987). The art therapist supports the individual making the drum in order for the individual to move through the emotionally charged experience and gain insight and therapeutic growth (Kramer 2001).

The drumming of the completed drum allows for kinesthetic energy to be part of the sublimation process and form a positive reframe for hitting an object. The playing of the drum allows for modification of negative behaviour, with the goal of improving affect (Kramer 2001). Through the therapeutic environment of the art studio and the drum circle, the art therapist supports the client in the efforts to express emotions and release highly charged impulses in a therapeutic, effective and productive manner. The support of the art therapist (assisting in choosing art materials and facilitating the drum circle) is vital in order for the therapeutic expression of emotion. An individual may not have adequate skills to express impulses and emotions and may experience emotional distress leading to negative outcomes without the assistance and guidance of the trained art therapist (Kramer 2001). The art making of the drum and the expressive participation within a facilitated drum circle, led by a therapist, allow for release of the energy and content of the unconscious drives in a healthy, constructive and socially acceptable form (Kramer 2001).

Object relations theory

Object relations theory evolved from Freudian theories that integrate the internal and unconscious drives of the individual, while internalizing the external influences from objects. Freud described the terminology of object as something that offers satisfaction to the need originating from an inner drive (Corey 1996; Goldenberg & Goldenberg 2008). Frequently, that object is a caregiver or individual of importance (Corey 1996; Goldenberg & Goldenberg 2008). According to Corey (1996), "Object relations are interpersonal relationships as they are represented intrapsychically" (p.81). It is through the interrelationships with objects that the infant or child will form attachments that profoundly influence their personality development and self-concept (Corey 1996). Attachment is the emotional connection that develops between an infant and the primary caregiver (Goldenberg & Goldenberg 2008). Winnicott (2005) credits the nurturing environment and caregiver as the deciding factors in the ability of the child to develop attachment.

The basic tenets of object relations theory include a focus on the examination of the relationship between self and the others (Goldenberg & Goldenberg 2008). Within human beings, there is an instinctual need to connect, form attachments and establish relationships with people (Dissanayake 1995; Goldenberg & Goldenberg 2008; Van der Kolk 2014). The determining factor of personality arises from the quality of the relationship between the infant and the primary caregiver. The relationship between the child and the primary caregiver forms the template for later adult relationships (Goldenberg & Goldenberg 2008).

Margaret Mahler was a pediatrician who studied the development of children and believed "progression from a symbiotic relationship with a maternal figure toward separation and individuation" held greater significance in the developmental process of children than that of the Oedipus complex that Freud proposed (Corey 1996, p.82). Mahler felt that the period of child development from birth to age three, along with the child's interactions and subsequent relationship with the primary caregiver, were the determining factors in the molding of the personality of the child. The psychological development of the child begins with fusion with the caregiver, evolves to separation between the caregiver and the self, and eventually leads to individuation and development of a concept of an individualized self (Corey 1996). The period of developing attachment and then progressing to individuation is of great significance and has a profound effect on later relationships. Mahler proposed the theory that the relationships of an adult are based in a deep desire to reconnect and reenact the first relationship stemming from the relationship with the primary caregiver, known as the object (Corey 1996).

Normal infantile autism

Mahler termed the stage of development within the first month of a child's life as normal infantile autism (Corey 1996). The child is driven by physical needs and is unable to recognize a separate self from that of the primary caregiver, most often the mother. The child is not able to synthesize the individual parts of the caregiver into a cohesive entity (Corey 1996). If the child's needs are consistently met, then the child will experience a blissful state of oneness with the caregiver (Corey 1996). During this period, a child is unable to exercise control of the relationship with the caregiver. Should the caregiver be unable to provide a nurturing environment, the child may experience frustration. Because of the child's limited development level, the child is unable to reconcile the nurturing and non-nurturing aspects of the caregiver. The child will split the experiences into good object, or the satisfying and nurturing caregiver, and bad object, or the non-nurturing caregiver (Corey 1996).

The good object provides the child with a sense of being loved and succeeds in making the child develop positive feeling in regard to self. The bad object is a source of frustration and results in feelings of being unloved developing within the child (Corey 1996). The child with the non-nurturing caregiver will experience feelings of anger and frustration while also possessing a desire to obtain love. These splits will become elements of the child's personality construct (Goldenberg & Goldenberg 2008). A good or bad introject results from the child's internalization of emotions related to the good and bad object (Goldenberg & Goldenberg 2008). If an individual is unable to demonstrate an organized sense of self, as a result of splitting and bad introjects, then the individual may demonstrate pathology (Corey 1996).

Symbiosis

The second stage of development, within object relations theory, is symbiosis (Corey 1996). Symbiosis begins at approximately three months of life and can last until the eighth month (Corey 1996). During this time period and stage, the child experiences dependence upon the caregiver and requires a great deal of "emotional attunement" from them for the satisfaction and gratification of needs (Corey 1996, p.83).

At approximately four months old the child enters the separation-individuation phase of development (Corey 1996). This is a time when the child begins to differentiate themselves from the caregiver, or object, and realizes separateness exists between oneself and the caregiver (Robbins 1998). The child is learning object constancy through the use of a transitional object (Winnicott 2005). The child has formed attachments with objects that act to soothe the child, such as a stuffed animal or blanket. These objects act to help the child establish a sense of separateness from the caregiver (Winnicott 2005). Winnicott (2005) states that "[t]he object represents the infant's transition from a state of being merged with the mother to a state of being in relation to the mother as something outside and separate" (pp.19–20). The child still requires the caregiver to provide support and validation, while being recognized as a discrete entity (Robbins 1998; Winnicott 2005).

Ambivalence

This is a time of ambivalence for the child resulting from the desire to gain independence and the continued need for dependence on the caregiver for survival (Corey 1996). The child must be allowed to physically explore their independence and environment and be welcomed upon their return; meanwhile, the caregiver provides a healthy mirror for the child's independence in order for the child to develop a healthy sense of self and positive self-esteem (Corey 1996). The development period lasts until the child is approximately three years old, during which time the child is developing object constancy and a sense of identity (Corey 1996; Robbins 1987). It is theorized that the child will be able to comprehend the world and individuals in a more holistic manner without splitting experiences into simple good or bad categories and has the ability to deal with ambivalence (Robbins 1998).

Object relations theory hypothesizes that it is imperative for the child to differentiate self from the caregiver (Corey 1996). The child must learn to idealize others and develop pride in their own abilities, which is learned through effective mirroring of the caregiver and by having the child's needs adequately met. Otherwise, the child may develop narcissistic personality disorder and poor self-esteem (Corey 1996) Corey (1996) states that "Narcissistic Personality Disorder is characterized by a grandiose and exaggerated sense of self-importance and an exploitative attitude towards others, which serve the function of masking a frail self-concept" (p.83). Individuals with this disorder seek attention and often have what is considered as an exaggerated or intensified degree of self-absorption in addition to a strong need to be admired by others. Narcissistic individuals are exploitative in interrelationships, while possessing a sense of emptiness that cannot be abated (Corey 1996).

The child is at risk of developing borderline personality disorder as a result of being unsuccessful in navigating the separation stage (Corey 1996). This is often the result of rejection and inadequate emotional support from the primary caregiver as the child attempts to separate and develop a sense of individuation (Corey 1996). People diagnosed with borderline personality disorder are "characterized by instability, irritability, self-destructive acts, impulsive anger and extreme mood shifts" (Corey 1996, pp.83–84). Individuals with this disorder are described as possessing labile mood and struggling with a sense of self-identity; they have difficulty understanding others, have poor impulse control and are incapable of tolerating real or imagined abandonment (APA 2013). Object relations theory posits that it is advantageous for the child to simultaneously experience a sense of independence along with a sense of attachment, thereby forming the foundation of a positive self-image and an ability to regard others with positive regard (Corey 1996).

Freud believed that transference and countertransference were essential aspects of the therapeutic relationship (Robbins 1987). These concepts and tools were carried over into object relations theory. As stated earlier, transference comprises the attitudes, emotions and perceptions that a client carries and projects upon the therapeutic relationship, or more precisely the therapist (Robbins 1987). Countertransference is the result of transference. Transference may act to emote emotions or actions within the therapist and may influence how the therapist responds to the client (Robbins 1987). Object relations theory utilizes transference as a means to provide insight into the developmental level of individuation and self-concept of the client (Robbins 1987).

Psychodynamic theorists focus on bringing unconsciousness into conscious awareness (Robbins 1987). Object relations theorists are not focused on the unconsciousness of the client. The main objective in object relations theory "is to move from partial object-relatedness, where the world is perceived as a good breast versus bad breast, to full object-relatedness" (Robbins 1987, p.26). Therapeutic treatment within object relations theory addresses modifying the individual's self-concepts from grandiose ideations to acceptance of human fallibilities, while revealing inappropriate self-concept structures that conceal fears of abandonment and loss (Robbins 1987).

Object relations theory and art therapy

Within the object relations model, the therapeutic relationship between the client and therapist acts to facilitate transference and countertransference to assist the client in navigating the processes of differentiation and individuation. The role of the therapist is one of openness in order to "mirror, complement, or confront the various internal representations" of the client (Robbins 1987, p.27). Communication based in empathy provides the connection that works to identify, understand and address defense mechanisms displayed by the client (Robbins 1987). Winnicott (2005) instructs the therapist to utilize art and play as a means to build transitional space, or a safe environment that acts as a bridge, between the client and the art. The art subsequently becomes the transitional object or other within the therapeutic experience. Through art, the client's self-concept and attachment to the object can be expressed within the image and symbols created (Winnicott 2005).

The role of the art therapist is to facilitate "primary creativity, or the early illusion of the infant that the world is his and that he can maintain a blissful state of oneness" (Robbins 1987, pp.27–28). Robbins (1987) refers to aesthetics as the process of "making the inanimate animate, giving form to diffuse energy or ideas, breathing life into sterile communication" (p.22). It is through the conveyance of truth via the aesthetic experience that the image becomes art (Robbins 1987). The art therapist employs creative aesthetics in order to restructure self-concepts while encouraging individuation and differentiation (Robbins 1987).

Winnicott (2005) explains that play is a vehicle to growth, health, communication and the development of social relationships. Play requires a space that exists neither inside of the child nor in the external world (Winnicott 2005). Play occurs in a space, often referred to as transitional space, that is between the caregiver and the child; dependent upon the environment created within the relationship between the child and the primary caregiver (Winnicott 2005). Within the transitional space, an individual is capable of reimagining the external world, objects and difficulties through the implementation of play, dreams and imagination (Winnicott 2005). Winnicott (2005) writes that "[i]t is in playing and only in playing that the individual child or adult is able to be creative and to use the whole personality, and it is only in being creative that the individual discovers self" (pp.72–73).

Creativity is the ability to approach the external world with hope and trust, for without creativity an individual is forced to live a life of compliance; and a life of compliance may not prove to be worth living (Winnicott 2005). The art therapist works to establish a space between the individual and the therapist that is founded in an experience filled with empathy, trust, positive mirroring and acceptance of the need for fusion and separateness (Robbins 1987). Through the effective use of transitional space and transitional objects based in art or play, a reimagining of reality is possible. Play and creativity offer the possibility of therapeutic change and growth (Winnicott 2005).

The therapeutic relationship is the key to therapeutic healing within the object relations model. The therapist is transparent within the interaction with the client through mirroring and praising appropriate behavior and affect as well as confronting other less desired behavior. The therapist builds a relationship with the client through empathy with the therapeutic space, or transitional space, that offers acceptance and understanding of the client's defenses (Robbins 1987). The therapist must be responsive to all the verbal and nonverbal communication provided by the client and be skilled in holding the space that bridges both subjective and objective realities (Robbins 1987). It is within this transitional space that the client is free to find expression through art, metaphor and play. The therapist and the art act to hold this space and reflect back the inappropriate or pathological states to the client. This allows for an exploration to discover a novel approach to integrate and incorporate therapeutic change and develops healthy forms of attachment and individuation (Robbins 1987).

Object relations theory and drumming

Art and drumming offer possibilities for transitional objects, transitional space and play (Mank 2019; Robbins 1987; Winnicott 2005). The therapeutic relationship offers potential for play through art in the form of painting a drum and creating a symbol of self upon the drum (Mank 2019). The symbol of self creates an object that is representative of the individual and yet separate from the individual (Schaverien 1992). The transitional object, or drum, then allows for exploration through playing within a supported environment of a facilitated drum circle. Individuals are supported by the drumming community and are offered opportunities to explore, play individually and then rejoin the drumming group. These exercises within the facilitated drum circle model key components of the object relations model to help restructure personality and attachment (Robbins 1987; Winnicott 2005).

Through playing a drum, which represents self, the individual is allowed to experiment with a new manner of being within the drumming community. The therapist, acting as a facilitator, and the drumming group within the structure of the drum circle, support the individual through rhythm and movement (Donovan 2015; Mank 2019; Stevens 2012, 2017). Appropriate behavior is mirrored back to the individual through positive reinforcement, building a stronger self-esteem and sense of attachment (Kossak 2015). The drum circle becomes the holding space, or transitional space, that allows for play through rhythm, auditory and visual stimulation, with energy that acts as a bridge between subjective and objective realities, or "primary and secondary process levels," allowing for therapeutic growth and change (Robbins 1987, p.28). It is within this creative space, while utilizing a transitional object, that the individual may find the blissful state of oneness and then move between levels of consciousness in a state of play (Robbins 1987). This state of play is similar to a meditative state and allows for openness to images and symbols while dissolving a sense of time and space (Robbins 1987). Within this transitional space, the individual can experience different energy levels while utilizing both processing levels to explore attachment and individuation via an "aesthetic response" (Robbins 1987, p.28).

Object relations theory with art therapy and drumming allow for exploration through rhythm and form, establishing an aesthetic experience that is based in attachment (Robbins 1987). The individual is allowed to experiment with fusion, separateness and individuation through the kinesthetic and visual experience of art, music and movement within the drum circle. The holding space is the circle, and the facilitator and drummers act as caregivers who reflect back appropriate behavior while allowing for processing on primary and secondary levels (Kossak 2015; Robbins 1987). Within this transitional space, the individual is allowed and encouraged to play and find alternative ways of being that can be utilized outside of the therapeutic space (Kossak 2015; Mank 2019; Winnicott 2005).

Attachment theory

Bowlby (1982) studied the relationships between the primary caregiver and young children under their care. The primary caregiver has influence over a child's ability to attach to others throughout the lifespan of the child. An infant develops an attachment style that is the product of the relationship between the caregiver and that infant (Bretherton 1992). The relationship developed between the child and the primary caregiver is one of reciprocity and depends upon the sensitivity and attunement of the caregiver to the various needs of the child (Bradley & Cafferty 2001). If the caregiver provides encouragement for a child to explore the environment, and that child is supported and praised upon return, then the child has a greater probability of developing a secure attachment style. The primary caregiver embodies a secure base, or sense of safety, to the child, which then provides the child with the confidence to explore the environment. The child is then free to return to the caregiver for reassurance, encouragement and praise (Bowlby 1982; Bretherton 1992). The secure base offers comfort in stressful times for the child. Mary Ainsworth built upon the research that Bowlby began on attachment (Bretherton 1992). Ainsworth invented the assessment entitled "Strange Situation" in order to study and identify the specific attachment style of the child with the primary caregiver (Bretherton 1992). Within the Strange Situation assessment, a child demonstrating secure attachment displayed emotions that indicated a level of distress at the departure of the primary caregiver. Once the primary caregiver had departed, the child with a secure attachment freely explored the environment, interacted with the various individuals in the specific room, and was welcoming to the primary caregiver upon return (Bretherton 1992).

In addition to secure attachment style, Ainsworth identified two more attachment styles within the Strange Situation research (Bretherton 1992). Anxious-avoidant attachment depicts a style of attachment of a child who displays a minor amount of emotion in response to the departure of the primary caregiver from the room. These children with anxious-avoidant attachment styles did not explore the environment after the caregiver left the room, and continued to display little emotion even when the primary caregiver returned to the room. It is believed that the lack of emotion displayed concealed the true level of distress the children may have experienced (Bretherton 1992).

A child who exhibits a sense of anxiousness prior to the caregiver leaving the room, and then behaves in a helpless manner while separated from the caregiver, and continues to display emotional distress and clingy behavior upon the caregiver's return, is thought to possess an anxious-resistant attachment (Bretherton 1992). Ainsworth believed that the attachment styles of secure, anxious-avoidant and anxious-resistant characterize a model or template. This template acts as a guide that informs and directs the formation of all future relationships throughout the entire lifespan of the person (Bretherton 1992).

Gillath and colleagues (2009) posit that individuals develop several attachment styles and that attachment styles are a state rather than a fixed trait. The attachment state exhibited is in response to the specific situation, relationship or event an individual is currently experiencing. Individuals may change their state of attachment as a result of experiences throughout their lifespan—for example, loss of a loved one, roles in society, and levels of independence (Bradley & Cafferty 2001).

Older adults often experience an increased sense of vulnerability as a result of age-related decline and chronic illness (Bradley & Cafferty 2001). Attachment style and caregiving relationships are of greater importance in later life (Bradley & Cafferty 2001). The adult child of an aging parent requiring care may experience an increase in protective feelings and actions in response to the strong sense of attachment to the aging parent. A greater sense of empathy for the aging parent is often the response experienced within the adult child providing care. The aging parent's attachment style has a great influence over the aging parent's emotional and behavioral reaction to chronic illness and the increased need for care (Bradley & Cafferty 2001). The attachment style of both the parent and child is an important variable that influences the response to the increased sense of vulnerability of the older adult or parent. Psychotherapy and the expressive arts have the potential to improve functioning, provide comfort and influence attachment style while addressing the levels of distress and vulnerability of the older adult (Gillath *et al.* 2009; Mank 2019; Rogers 1993).

Mirroring, attachment and neurological development

As previously stated, the first three years of life are of considerable importance as a result of the neurological and psychological development and maturation occurring during this time period (Bowlby 1982; Chapman 2014; Schore & Schore 2008). The optimal caregiver/child relationship is founded upon a secure attachment that is cultivated through the caregiver's adeptness in identifying, responding and attuning to the profound changes in the "infant's bodily-based internal states of central and autonomic arousal" (Schore & Schore 2008). The degree of attunement by the caregiver to the child's ever-changing needs directly affects the development of the child's central nervous system (CNS) and autonomic nervous system (ANS) and impacts the child's attachment style and psychological development (Bowlby 1982; Schore & Schore 2008; Winnicott 2005).

A child who is exposed to inadequate or poor attunement by the caregiver will suppress behaviors that are indicative of attachment and comfort-based needs and may learn to fear expressing basic needs related to care (Baylin & Hughes 2016). The brain of the child receiving poor care will develop differently than that of a child with an attuned caregiver. A child with an attuned caregiver will develop neurological circuitry and a neurotransmitter system that encourages the development of attachment with a caregiver (Baylin & Hughes 2016).

Through the interactions between the child and the attuned caregiver there are often times of eye-to-eye contact (Baylin & Huges 2016; Chapman 2014; Kossak 2015). Mirroring is evident during continued eye contact between the child and caregiver where the caregiver mimics the facial expressions and affect of the child (Chapman 2014; Kossak 2015; Winnicott 2005; Wright 2009). If a secure attachment is achieved along with mirroring during the critical period of the first three years of life, then there is a high probability that the child will develop a strong and effective sense of self (Stott 2017; Winnicott 2005). It is through the mirroring process that the child witnesses their own experience reflected upon the face of their caregiver (Stott 2017). The inability of the child to develop and experience a reciprocal relationship with the primary caregiver results in construction and development of pathological psychological defenses as an attempt to compensate for the lack of connection and secure attachment to the primary caregiver (Stott 2017).

Recent studies have raised awareness of the vital connection between the mind and the body (Chapman 2014; Kossak 2015; Van der Kolk 2014; Wright 2009). Throughout the progression of attachment, the caregiver and the child have interactions founded in the somatic senses. The five senses associated with the reciprocal interactions of the caregiver/child relationship act to stimulate the child's neurological development and influence attachment (Chapman 2014). The developing child absorbs information primarily through the somatic senses (Baylin & Hughes 2016). The child who receives adequate care from an attuned caregiver will create a bias, in the neural development of the sensory system within the brain, toward stimuli that indicate safety. On the other hand, the child who does not receive adequate care will develop neurological circuitry biased towards identifying stimuli that indicate danger (Baylin & Hughes 2016).

It is during the first two years of life that the neural circuit wiring of the orbital prefrontal cortex is forming and developing (Schore 2000). Bowlby (1982) asserts that, during this same time period, attachment is established, suggesting a connection between the somatic senses, attachment style and neurological development of the brain (Bowlby 1982; Chapman 2014; Wright 2009).

Research suggests that the relationship between the client and the therapist holds the potential to affect neurological changes within the brain of the client (Kossak 2015). It is theorized that the mirror neuron system within the brain of an individual is activated and stimulated during, and as a result of, reciprocal relationships. Within a reciprocal relationship where one individual experiences either an auditory or visual stimulation, the activation of the mirror neurons occurs in one individual. The other individual will experience a sympathetic response to the first individual's mirror neuron activation (Kossak 2015). Within the realm of a therapeutic alliance or relationship, the mirror neuron activation within the brain of the client will initiate a sympathetic response within the therapist (Kossak 2015).

The mirror neuron system allows an individual to comprehend the emotions and behavior of other human beings as an "embodied being" (Kossak 2015, p.104.) The ability to understand the personal lived experience of other human beings is defined as "embodied empathy" or "attunement" (Kossak 2015, p.104). The mirror neuron system is formed in the brain of the infant as a result of the caregiver's attention and attunement to the infant's needs and state of emotions (Kossak 2015; Stott 2017; Wright 2009).

The expressive arts offer corresponding experiences to that of a caregiver's attunement to an infant (Kossak 2015; Wright 2009). The creation and witnessing of the expressive arts provides opportunities to evoke emotion and empathy that emulate those of the artist, which, in turn, stimulate an embodied empathetic response, or attunement, between the individual involved and the specific art form (Kossak 2015). The attunement established within the expressive arts provides opportunities for the formation of a therapeutic alliance between the therapist and the client.

The therapeutic alliance, which is constructed through immersion in the expressive arts, promotes spontaneity and an awareness of the overt and hidden aspects of self for members of this therapeutic group

(Kossak 2015). The attention and attunement to embodied awareness, along with changes of consciousness, allow for a safe space for exploration and risk taking with possibilities of meaning making, as experienced within the therapeutic alliance (Kossak 2015). This therapeutic, safe place based in creativity and therapeutic growth, or change, is called transitional space (Winnicott 2005). Within the transitional space of the therapeutic alliance the client has the opportunity to explore and discover meaning whilst experiencing the emotional support of the therapist in which the expressive arts are engaged (Winnicott 2005).

Attachment theory and drumming

The application and employment of object relations and attachment theories combined with the expressive arts, as facilitated within a therapeutic milieu and within a therapeutic alliance, has shown success in the alteration and reduction of pathological coping mechanisms and personality traits (Rogers 1993; Schaverien 1992). Object relations and attachment theories have determined the significance of cultivating positive and productive relationships, constructing secure attachment styles through attunement and a therapeutic alliance in order to experience therapeutic growth and change (Bowlby 1982; Kossak 2015; Schaverien 1992; Winnicott 2005). Mank (2019) conducted a research study that employed the expressive arts, object relations theory and attachment therapy in order to establish and maintain a therapeutic milieu, attain attunement and offer opportunities for play while discovering new approaches to cope with the transitions associated with the aging process. The study indicated that art and drumming, within the therapeutic alliance and safe milieu, significantly changed attachment styles to one of secure attachment for participants who resided independently in the community. Mank (2019) determined that the drumming group had potential for the participants to form attunement and attachment to one another and to the facilitator by means of play and exploration. The drumming aspect of the study modeled appropriate behavior while participants developed social and musical skills and created a sense of belonging to fellow members of the research group as well as to the entire group and activity (Mank 2019).

Conclusion

The psychodynamic theory of sublimation allows individuals to redirect socially inappropriate energy to more acceptable behavior through art and drumming. The role of the therapist is to support the client through selection of art materials and understanding of the symbolic meaning within a safe and controlled environment that allows for manageable expression of emotions (Kramer 1972; Naumburg 1973; Rubin 1987). Object relations theory, along with attachment theory, offers opportunities for the restructuring of pathological coping skills and behavior while working toward secure attachment through the therapeutic alliance and through art and drumming (Bowlby 1982; Gillath *et al.* 2009; Kossak 2015; Mank 2019; Rogers 1993; Schaverien 1992; Winnicott 2005). Through the formation and utilization of a therapeutic milieu and alliance, the therapist offers the client opportunities to play, explore and work toward therapeutic growth and change (Winnicott 2005).

CHAPTER 3

Signs and Symbols

Dissanayakhe (1995) writes that the creation of art has continued throughout the ages and is evident in nearly all cultures and societies across time. Art and ancient symbols have existed for thousands of years although the purpose and symbolic meaning may not be concretely known. There are several theories that do exist which may explain the purpose of the ancient art or symbols. What is known is that "art seems to answer some basic human need that transcends the particular expectations and purposes that any given society assigns it" (Haslam 1997, p.2). The visual arts continue to transform and evolve according to the needs of the modern world and society at large (Haslam 1997).

During the most recent time of redefinition of the visual arts, art therapy has emerged and has provided a means for therapeutic growth, healing and change (Haslam 1997). Art therapy is founded upon theories originally proposed by both Freud and Jung along with shamanism and man's need for artistic expression (Dissanayake 1995; Haslam 1997).

Haslam (1997) discusses archeological finds of pigments within pottery and cave paintings in Europe that are believed to be 150,000–200,000 years old. The images created in the caves were acted upon repeatedly by the society that created them as a form of ritualistic behavior within an organized spiritual system (Haslam 1997). The caves and the paintings are elements of a spiritual practice that held significance as "ceremonial sanctuaries or sacred shrines" (Haslam 1997, p.4).

It is believed that the first shamans were artists and that they utilized spirituality, ritual and artistic expression as forms of communication and tools for healing (Haslam 1997). The key component of shamanism is the ability of the shaman to place themselves within a trance, or altered state of consciousness, through the use of the expressive arts (Haslam 1997). The shaman often uses chants, drumming or dancing to achieve an altered state of consciousness. The spiritual and ritualistic practices of shamans were, and still are, for healing purposes and to align the patient with, and to, the universe. The paintings the shamans created were composed of powerful symbols that acted in a manner to empower the shamans and participants within the ritual practice of spirituality (Haslam 1997).

There are more archeological discoveries that include animal bones, human bones and skulls which were preserved and cared for in a ceremonial fashion in Europe, the Middle East and China. Some of these bones were those of homo erectus and the Neanderthals and are approximately 500,000 years old (Haslam 1997). The ceremonial manner in which the bones were arranged and preserved represent the origins of spirituality in humans and suggests a consciousness within these individuals (Haslam 1997). The spirituality of the early humans suggests that they were capable of abstract thought, possessed a sense of time and space, and were capable of communication of concepts prior to "the development of fully articulated speech" (Haslam 1997, p.3).

Langer (1957) noted that the mind of human beings is active and does not turn off or stop, even during sleep. The human mind actively constructs ideas and thoughts. Man's use of signs and symbols is the primary indication of abstract thought and of an intelligent mind (Langer 1957). The ability to create and utilize symbols is a distinguishing feature that separates humans from all other species on earth (Wilson 1985).

Signs and symbols are ubiquitous in modern human life. Langer (1957) defines signs as things that confirm the existence of an object, an experience, an occasion or a condition that exist in time, albeit past, present or future (Langer 1957). A sign is a "stand-in" for or a representation of something concrete that indicates something specific and does not convey deeper meaning (Morrell 2011; Wilson 1985). Langer (1957) believed that the comprehension and use of signs was the beginning of the expression of the mind of man (Langer 1957).

Langer (1957) theorizes that symbolism evolved from the propitious utilization of signs. Morrell (2011) specifies that "humans use a system of signs to communicate about both concrete and abstract concepts."

A symbol conveys abstract thoughts and concepts about the object being denoted in the symbol (Langer 1957). The creation of symbols is a basic process within the mind of man and is crucial to thought (Langer 1957). Speech and language are symbols that communicate concepts related to objects and convey meaning (Langer 1957). Isserow (2013) concurred with the theory that the essence of humanity is founded upon man's ability to form symbols, thereby creating possibilities of communication between human beings.

Jung and von Franz (1964) define a symbol as "a term, name or even a picture that may be familiar in daily life, yet that possesses specific connotations in addition to its conventional and obvious meaning" (Part 1, Section 1, para. 2). A symbol suggests something more than the known and unmistakable meaning (Jung & von Franz 1964). Jung and von Franz (1964) include art and images as symbolic form when greater meaning is implied than that which is overtly observed in the visual representation.

There is a limit to man's ability to consciously understand or fully comprehend ideas, objects or concepts (Jung & von Franz 1964). For this reason, man invariably creates symbols to represent ideas or concepts that are not fully understood or known (Jung & von Franz 1964). Haslam (1997) explains that symbols are rife with diverse meanings and act as a point of convergence. If one were to strip the symbol of all its meaning, then the symbol would become a sign and be unable to convey, contain or become a source for discovery of conscious and unconscious material (Haslam 1997).

Barash (2008) discusses the theories of Cassirer in regard to symbols. Symbols occupy a duality of existence in that a symbol is an object (for example, an image on canvas) that is capable of conveying meaning on a universal level and is specific to the culture in which it was created (Barash 2008). Symbols traverse the realms of sensory knowledge and that of spiritual awareness. Symbols are able to direct awareness to something greater that occurs in nature, culture or in mythical realms (Barash 2008).

Naumberg viewed the client's artwork as symbolic; it conveyed meaning that was known only to the artist (Rubin 1987). The art evokes the essence of the thing being portrayed in the symbol and often contains latent meaning (Edwards 1987). Art can be created in reflection and as a meditative process in response to the original art, or symbol, as a mechanism to delve deeper to reach the unconscious and understand meaning contained in the art (Allen 1995). Wilson (1987) states that through the creation of art, or symbols, unconscious information can be brought into conscious understanding that acts to create therapeutic growth and change. The art therapist acts to support the client through the discovery of symbolic meaning contained in the artwork (Rubin 1987).

Symbols and culture

The preponderant use of symbols through artistic and ritualistic practices sanctioned social customs that encouraged personal and group resolutions to problems while advocating cohesion of group identity and stability (Haslam 1997). Dissanayake (1999) noted that, through ritual and making special, individuals became united and formed cohesive groups that held greater probability for survival. Symbols contain the ability to unite individuals through cultural practice and communication, thereby holding greater connectivity between members of the group and offering possibilities for unity, survival and understanding (Haslam 1997).

Holland and Valsiner (1988) discuss the theories of Vygotsky that pertain to symbols as mediating devices. A mediating device is a developmental process where symbols are originally used with the social domain of a culture and are then incorporated into a mental function. Humans use symbols to organize and structure thought processes of the mind. Through the organization of symbols within the thought process, an individual is able to modify their own mental and emotional state. The modification of mental and emotional states through symbols, or mediating devices, becomes a pivotal point in the evolution of humans (Holland & Valsiner 1988).

Symbols serve as tools to develop self-control of both cognition and emotions, thereby affecting social and cultural environments, and contribute to collective understanding (Holland & Valsiner 1988). The evocative nature of symbols expands in relation to the function the symbol plays in the development of cognition and emotional content within a culture or society. The symbol becomes internalized within the individual and becomes representative of a society's value system, which is composed of a variety of thoughts and emotions (Holland

& Valsiner 1988). Symbols represent the internalized organization of cultural values and knowledge.

Jung and von Franz (1964) identify the need for symbolic images in religion as being due to a lack of knowledge and limitations in the understanding of concepts by the general public. Religious art is not the only medium in which symbols are found: "Man also produces symbols unconsciously and spontaneously, in the form of dreams" (Jung & von Franz 1964, Part 1, Section 1, para. 4). Within dreams, the unconscious portion of any experience is divulged through symbolic form, although the content is not revealed directly (Jung & von Franz 1964).

Dream imagery

Because of the advancement of modern technology and the knowledge gained, many ideas and concepts have been stripped of emotional energy (Jung & von Franz 1964). Through symbolic image within dreams, an individual has little choice but to pay attention to the image and message (Jung & von Franz 1964). It is through the symbolic language of dreams that an individual's "psychological balance" is restored (Jung & von Franz 1964, Part 1, Section 3, para. 29).

Archetypes

Although dream content is rich in symbolic images and meaning, dreams are not the only resource for symbols. Jung and von Franz (1964) write that symbols appear "in all kinds of psychic manifestations" (Part 1, Section 4, para. 2). Jung and von Franz (1964) theorize that symbols are often religious in nature, instinctual, mythic and beyond the regulation of consciousness. Man is subject to instinctual actions and urges just as other creatures are influenced by instinct. Man has inherited collective thought paradigms, known as archetypes, which are perceived as impulses, instinct, or forces that act to guide the unconscious (Jung & von Franz 1964). Archetypes are not stagnant and point to things that are outside the complete comprehension of the conscious mind (Jung & von Franz 1964). The inherited knowledge of archetypes is components of the collective unconscious that all humans possess knowledge of and to which there is access (Jung & von Franz 1964).

In order to understand the symbols within the dream content, it is imperative to look at the gestalt, or wholeness, of the symbol, which includes the collective unconscious, archetypal images and the individual who produced the symbol (Jung & von Franz 1964). Jung and von Franz (1964) define natural symbols as originating from the unconscious and epitomize adaptations of archetypal images from the earliest civilizations. Cultural symbols are used in religions and have evolved over time to become "collective images accepted by civilized society" (Jung & von Franz 1964, Part 1, Section 8, para. 1). Therefore, it is necessary to determine whether symbolic images are related to the personal experience of the individual or whether the symbol originates from the collective unconscious based in archetypal imagery (Jung & von Franz 1964).

Connection to symbols

Archetypal imagery contains emotional energy due to the symbolic meaning and therefore acts as a dynamic force (Jung & von Franz 1964). It is through the emotional energy of the archetypal image that a connection is formed with the individual: "Archetypes are pieces of life itself – images that are integrally connected to the living individual by the bridge of emotions" (Jung & von Franz 1964, Part 1, Section 8, para. 17). The connection between archetypal imagery and emotions actuates a compelling force that facilitates a connection to the primitive self, or psyche, when in relationship with an individual (Jung & von Franz 1964).

The dynamic force of a symbol offers potential for connection and communication on an interpersonal and intrapersonal level (Isserow 2013). The symbol can hold rich and complex meaning that provides an alternative perspective for the viewer. The binding factor between the viewer and the symbol is the emotional connection that unifies the viewer to the symbol (Haslam 1997). Therapeutic transformation is dependent upon the artist's and/or viewer's sense of unity with the symbol and the unconscious material it holds (Haslam 1997). It is through the communal experience of the conveyance of symbolic meaning that therapeutic change and growth are possible (Isserow 2013).

Symbolic meaning is not static and is often in a state of change or flow (Haslam 1997). The variance of meaning of a symbol has the potential to transform the individual who possesses a connection to the symbol (Haslam 1997). The symbol has the ability to provide access to the psyche, thereby providing information and knowledge that was previously unknown on a conscious level. This ability to access unconscious material through symbolic form provides an opportunity for therapeutic growth (Haslam 1997).

The cyclical nature of the internalization process offers opportunities for identification of symbolic meaning, review of unconscious information and reintegration of the knowledge gained through the processing of symbols, which opens possibilities for self-awareness, understanding and therapeutic change and growth (Haslam 1997). Haslam (1997) explains that the process of identifying with a symbol and incorporating it into one's sense of self is internalization. As an individual creates an artistic rendering of the symbol through art making, the process of externalization takes place. The symbol becomes a tangible object and occupies a concrete role in reality outside the mind of the individual. The symbol is now a separate entity from the individual, allowing for objective viewing and dialog. The material that was unconscious prior to externalization is now visible and available for review and for synthesis of knowledge through the process of internalization (Haslam 1997).

Langer (1957) postulates that human expression is not passive but is productive and dynamic. Symbols are used to establish and organize ideas, faith and knowledge. The power of the use of symbols resides in the ability to move from strictly sensory data to abstract thought and the expression of emotions. Langer (1957) believed that the fundamental expression of thought is through symbolization, which includes language in humans. Symbolization is the pivotal expression of the mental capacity of humans. Thought, as expressed in symbols, is a determining factor in the actualization of a mind within humans (Langer 1957).

Langer observed that symbolic meaning within art evoked emotional responses from the viewer (Julliard & Van Den Heuvel 1999). The artwork is a culmination of symbols that are founded upon ingrained tradition and a sequence of signs. Each piece of art is a unique and distinct symbol whose elements reside exclusively within the totality of the artwork (Julliard & Van Den Heuvel 1999). The emotional force experienced by the viewer of a particular piece of artwork is the result of the intuitively experienced emotion that is embodied in symbolic form. The artwork is essentially a visual symbol that is the emissary of a sensed concept, or idea, whose power is located in the conveyed meaning of the art piece itself. The meaning conveyed within the artwork, or symbol, is its own reality (Julliard & Van Den Heuvel 1999). The reality conveyed in the art is the focus of inquiry within art therapy.

Symbolic form within art therapy

Art therapy becomes a vehicle to reconstruct a lived experience into artistic form that allows others to observe and identify with the emotions of the artist's reality (Julliard & Van Den Heuvel 1999). Utilizing symbolic form to illuminate emotions and meaning expressed through artwork moves the experience from a cognitive level to a deeper, emotional level. The enlightenment that results allows the artist, or client, to fully experience emotions, thoughts and meaning encompassed within the reality depicted in the artwork (Julliard & Van Den Heuvel 1999). Art therapy has the capacity to reshape the emotional experience and reality of the client through the process of experiencing and understanding the emotional content of the artwork.

It should be noted that symbolic meaning is revealed through the art (Chapman 2014). Art materials, in conjunction with the artist, facilitate the creation of symbols and meaning that are beyond the limitations of verbal language. Through art and the symbolic form contained within the reality expressed in the art, meaning is conveyed and understood, and therapeutic growth is possible. Art becomes the messenger that conveys conscious, unconscious, social and cultural meaning (Allen 1995; Chapman 2014; Jung 1963).

Symbols, drum making and drumming

Mank (2019) found that the creation of a symbol of self that was painted on a drum after completing ten weeks of drumming acted as a tangible reminder of the individual's creativity by the other members of the drumming group. Creativity was evident through the improvised drum rhythms. However, the art image of the symbol of self that was created on a self-ascribed drum offered a visual reminder of creativity as well as conveying information about the participant to the rest of the group in addition to the creator of the symbol. Some members of the group created images related to their culture and country of origin while others painted images that were representative of a love of nature, their philosophy on life, a favorite pet, or that acted as a symbol of strength through difficult times. Each drum was unique and held symbolic meaning to the creator of the image while offering insight and information pertaining to the individual who created the symbol. The drum became the transitional object for the participant, who created the image and played the drum within the drum circle, offering the opportunity to play and explore in a therapeutic milieu and within a therapeutic alliance. Within the study, the participants learned more about the creativity and inner experience of the symbol creator through conversations pertaining to the symbol created on the drum. The participants of the study stated that the creation of the symbol of self and subsequent conversations, along with drumming, created a greater sense of belonging between the members of the group within the research study than prior to symbol creation (Mank 2019).

Conclusion

A symbol connotes something: an idea, a concept, a sense of spirituality or an emotion (Jung & von Franz 1964; Langer 1957). The creation of a symbol brings the intangible into the corporeal reality (Langer 1957). The self-concept of the individual is brought into reality through the creation of a symbol of self on the drum. This symbol offers glimpses of how the individual conceives of self. Through the ritual of drumming upon a transitional object, which is simultaneously both self and not self, an individual experiences a symbolic reconstruction or transformation that other mediums of expression cannot provide (Langer 1957; Mank 2019). The symbol evokes the concept of the individual, and the ritual induces cohesiveness within the drumming group that may lead to growth and change (Dissanayake 1995; Langer 1957; Winnicott 2005).

CHAPTER 4

Music and Music Therapy

Music is an integral part of human culture and daily life. It can be found cross-culturally and is believed to have existed for countless centuries of human existence (Bruscia 2014; Darnley-Smith & Patey 2003; Dissanayake 2000). Styles, content and compositions of music are unique to the culture, population and setting in which it is created, performed and appreciated (Darnley-Smith & Patey 2003). Music has the capability to offer comfort, create community and evoke emotion in the musician, composer and listener (Darnley-Smith & Patey 2003; Stevens 2012). Bruscia (2014) defines music as "the art of organizing sounds in time" (p.13). A broad definition of music includes sounds that are organized around a rhythm or melody (Darnley-Smith & Patey 2003). These sounds can be mechanical, vocal or instrumental (Darnley-Smith & Patey 2003).

There is difficulty in specifying the exact origin of music on account of its intrinsic temporal nature (Darnley-Smith & Patey 2003). However, there is evidence of preserved bone flutes, found in the domestic living areas of ruins and in caves in Europe, that are approximately 35,000 years old (Cook & British Museum 2013; Dissanayake 2000) It is believed that the utilization of sound for emotional expression began before verbal language existed in humans (Darnley-Smith & Patey 2003; Dissanayake 2000; Levitin 2016). Infants, who are preverbal, often respond to rhythm, vocal singing and play, indicating that verbal language is not required in order to have an emotional response or connection to music (Dissanayake 2000; Levitin 2016). Moreover, according to Friedman (2000), "Infants who receive steady, strong rhythmic messages through rocking with loving sounds from a caregiver, have quicker visual and auditory development" (p.24). The properties of music, and especially the musical property of rhythm, provide emotional response and connection that lead to healthy human development (Friedman 2000).

The elemental properties of music include rhythm, pitch, timbre and melody (Darnley-Smith & Patey 2003). Rhythm is defined as the duration of a group or series of notes and how these notes are unified into a pattern (Levitin 2016). Pitch refers to the frequency and location of a tone on a musical scale. Timbre is the distinguishing marker or feature of an instrument that differentiates one instrument from another, such as a piano from a flute, when playing the same note. Melody is a sequence of tones that are the most notable or memorable from a piece of music (Levitin 2016). It is the convergence of the aforementioned properties that combine and create an art and communication form known as music (Levitin 2016).

Music is a prominent, or ubiquitous, element in many cultures and provides a medium to unite the community by providing a vehicle in which to express thoughts, ideas and emotions, and to build cohesiveness within a community (Wanjala & Kebaya 2016). The music one listens to shapes one's sense of social and personal identity, especially among youth who are actively searching for, and are in the process of forming, a sense of identity. Historical references, culture and language may be incorporated within the musical piece or genre to connect with, inform and express opinions, which may lead to sociocultural identity construction within the listening audience. The musical artist provides a platform to articulate thoughts and to unite members of society through symbolic form within the musical expression, thereby affecting social change and identity within the listening audience (Wanjala & Kebaya 2016).

Historically and cross-culturally, humans have utilized music as a vehicle for social introduction and cohesion, thereby elevating the experience through ritual (Dissanayake 1995; Longhofer & Floersch 1993). Rites of passage, such as introducing an infant into the family and community, hunting, harvesting, marriage, death and battle, are rituals often accompanied with drumming and the arts to make the event special and meaningful (Bensimon, Amir & Wolf 2008; Dissanayake 1995; Longhofer & Floersch 1993). Through music a connection to history and traditions can be made while weaving the wisdom of the past into the present through playing traditional rhythms, dancing and singing (Longhofer & Floersch 1993).

A frequent topic of research is how various musical experiences may affect health and wellbeing of individuals in both clinical and ordinary life situations (Semenza 2018). Research studies have found that participants within a therapeutic milieu experience a greater sense of happiness, a reduction in anxiety, and benefit both physically and psychologically as a result of participating in the musical dosage. Experiencing music, within the context of coping with physical or mental illness, offers opportunities for reevaluation and perspective (Semenza 2018). Music can aid in distancing an individual from "the physical burden of disease" in addition to transforming the experience from one of disease to one of recovery by offering coping mechanisms and providing opportunity to exercise emotional regulation (Semenza 2018).

Identity and the expressive arts

The development and formation of a sense of self, or identity, is a flexible and evolving process that is the result of a response to life experiences, societal relationships, culture, roles and social values (McCaffrey Irish World Academy 2013; Stets & Burke 2000). Stets & Burke (2000) contend that "the self is reflexive in that it can take itself as an object and can categorize, or name itself in particular way" based upon societal and cultural classifications. It is through this form of social organization and classification that a personal identity, or identified sense of self, is forged. The social identity theory asserts there is a "reciprocal relationship between self and society" (Cinoglu & Arikan 2012). Culture and society provide the template for a social identity assumed by an individual (McClellan 2014). An identity cannot be formed without input and experiences from the culture and the society in which the individual perceives a sense of membership. A sense of self is based and founded upon the past and present relationships and experiences with significant others and the culture and society to which an individual expresses affinity (Cinoglu & Arikan 2012; McClellan 2014).

Identity theory depicts self-identity as a perception of self that is adopted and assumed by an individual based on the roles that they accept within society or the community in which they reside, or to which they feel a sense of belonging (Rise, Sheeran & Hukkelberg

2010). The self is defined as the "meanings and expectations" derived from a specific role that one chooses to integrate into one's value system, or standards, and which ultimately acts to direct and guide one's behavior (Rise *et al.* 2010). Subsequently, behavior is a direct result of the attitudes and values of self-selected, societal roles and the personal meanings derived from the assumption of those roles (Rise *et al.* 2010).

In order to fully understand oneself or others, an individual must "understand and investigate the society that took part" in the formation of the social identity of the individual (Cinoglu & Arikan 2012). Stets & Burke (2000) argue that the value of existence and what value is derived from performing tasks are the foundation of identity formation. The expressive arts have the potential to be a central component in the formation of identity. There is an "innate healing power of creative activity" that comprises a recognized sense of increased confidence, self-esteem and wellbeing as well as mastery (Archibald *et al.* 2010). The expressive arts provide a mechanism in which to develop and form an identity through the imaginative reality and symbolic meaning the expressive arts create via the performance and/or making of the specific art form (Archibald *et al.* 2010; Wanjala & Kebaya 2016).

Music and the expressive arts augment and elevate rituals, thereby providing possibilities for a sense of connection to others and to the divine (Dissanayake 1995, 2000). Rogers (1993) theorizes that through engagement of the expressive arts and allowing one art form to influence the next, a connection to universality, or something greater than oneself, is possible. Self-transcendence, or universality, offers the possibility to discover novel and unique aspects of self, create meaning and experience spirituality (Rogers 1993).

The implementation of music within a ritual exercise generates a contingency for self-transcendence, also described as a detached aesthetic experience, where an individual adopts a stance of openness and relinquishes control while allowing for a dissolution of boundaries for the purpose of experiencing the "flow of feeling" over the individual's personal sense of self (Dissanayake 1995, p.133). The aesthetic experience, consisting of a feeling of timelessness without a definitive sense of boundaries, provides the opportunity to reveal universal truths that may effectively unify individuals. Music acts as a vehicle to connect to, comprehend and internalize both the physical and spiritual planes, with opportunities to experience altered states of consciousness

(Rugenstein 2000). Connection to a sense of something greater than the self, via the arts and an altered state of consciousness, facilitates access to the unconscious and possibilities for insight and cathartic experiences, which may lead to greater knowledge of self (Jung 1963; Rugenstein 2000).

Music and mental health

Music has been identified as an agent of change in an individual's development of self (DeNora 2000; Rolvsjord & Stige 2015). Music directly expresses the values of a culture or society while influencing individuals on personal levels in regard to mood, spirituality, personality development and structure, and memory. DeNora (2000) writes that studies found participants were cognizant of personal needs in regard to informing and altering their own self-concept and sense of self.

Musical selection and listening have the capability to act to stabilize a sense of self within an individual, improve mood and maintain positive mental health (Semenza 2018). Self-selection of musical listening choices have been shown to reduce emotional reactions and physiological arousal responses to negative life stressors (Semenza 2018). Listening to self-selected musical choices, which are employed as a form of self-improvement or as a coping skill, has been shown to instill happiness, improve concentration and develop a positive sense of identity (Semenza 2018).

The ability to evaluate one's own emotions objectively is termed emotional reflexivity and acts to aid in emotional regulation (Semenza 2018). Both emotional regulation and emotional reflexivity are essential in attaining and maintaining positive mental health. Conscious selection of musical experiences to reflect upon emotions supports the reduction of stress and the subsequent negative effects of stress that manifest upon the body and mental health of the individual (Semenza 2018). It is through the reflection on one's own emotions objectively, with the regulation of emotions, that one may improve mental health within the context of ordinary life (Semenza 2018). Past childhood musical experiences provide salient experiences that increase the probability of utilizing music as a coping skill later in life to augment and contribute to wellbeing in adults (Semenza 2018). Utilizing music as a coping skill offers opportunity for reflection and emotional regulation, which are effective mechanisms in maintaining positive mental health (Semenza 2018).

Music therapy

The American Music Therapy Association (AMTA) defines music therapy as a health profession where music is utilized within the therapeutic relationship, between the music therapist and client, in order to address and respond to the social, physical, emotional or cognitive needs of the client (AMTA 2019). The clinical application of musical interventions is founded upon research and is evidence-based, specifically chosen and aimed to address predetermined goals and improve the wellbeing of the client (AMTA 2019; McCaffrey Irish World Academy 2013). The focus of music therapy includes assessing the strengths of the client and providing care through a multitude of treatments, including musical creation, vocal singing, movement or listening to music for the therapeutic purpose of improving or achieving the wellbeing of the client. Through music, emotional expression and communication are possible via verbal or nonverbal means. The music-based, therapeutic relationship identifies and builds upon strengths in the client to develop skills that are applicable to all domains in their life (AMTA 2019).

Music therapy is a contemporary profession in which there are specific requisite skills along with an understanding of a theoretical framework of knowledge and a dedication to music for the purpose of providing care and wellbeing to those in need (Darnley-Smith & Patey 2003). Music therapy is difficult to define because it is transdisciplinary in nature. The discipline of music therapy draws from, and is composed of, a fusion of music, therapy, psychology, the creative arts, the humanities, education, science and medicine, and has deep roots grounded in culture (Bruscia 2014; Darnley-Smith & Patey 2003; Stevens 2012; Wanjala & Kebaya 2016). Music therapy is founded on the construct that music is a language in its own right that contains meaning and is reciprocal in nature between the client and the music therapist (McCaffrey Irish World Academy 2013). Music therapy gives the client the opportunity to express emotions, identify and develop positive coping skills, and explore and resolve significant issues through the aesthetic experience of sound as supported and facilitated by a trained music therapist (Darnley-Smith & Patey 2003).

Music therapy is an aesthetic experience that is sound-based and therefore ear-centric (Darnley-Smith & Patey 2003). Music has the ability to convey a journey from conflict to resolution through the use of creativity, resulting in an instillation of meaning (Darnley-Smith & Patey 2003). Therapeutic and creative encounters with music engender beauty and deep satisfaction to provide meaning to life (Darnley-Smith & Patey 2003). Creating and listening to music, within the therapeutic relationship, promotes opportunities for emotional expression through rhythm, melody and lyrics that allow for subjectivity, objectivity, release and connection to assist in therapeutic change and to unite oneself with significant others and the greater community (Bruscia 2014; Darnley-Smith & Patey 2003; Wanjala & Kebaya 2016).

The music therapist is informed by a researched body of information and knowledge in order to serve the health-focused goals of the client within a therapeutic relationship grounded in music (Bruscia 2014). The role of the music therapist is to be supportive and empathetic to the life experience of the client while bearing witness to the journey of the client toward wellbeing (Bruscia 2014). The music therapist must maintain a stance of reflexivity (Bruscia 2014; Darnley-Smith & Patey 2003). Reflexivity entails a persistent and routine practice of self-awareness, evaluation and inquiry to identify beliefs, therapeutic approaches and to best serve the client (Bruscia 2014; Darnley-Smith & Patey 2003).

Darnley-Smith and Patey (2003) inform the reader that there are five ways of developing reflexivity: self-observation; self-inquiry; awareness; evaluation; supervision and consultation. The music therapist must conduct a continual process of self-observation, self-inquiry, awareness and evaluation within the session and throughout the therapeutic process, allowing for modification of treatment when necessary. The therapist must obtain supervision and consultation as necessary and throughout the course of therapy, all the while collaborating with the client (Darnley-Smith & Patey 2003).

There are four primary classifications of music therapy methods employed to achieve the goals of the client (Darnley-Smith & Patey 2003): improvisation, playing or singing previously recorded or pre-composed music, composition of novel music, and listening to pre-composed and previously recorded music. All categories assume that music is the principal medium in which music therapy occurs between the client and the music therapist. Music within the context of music therapy acts as a process, a mechanism and an outcome for the purpose of serving the needs of the client (Bruscia 2014).

Music therapy may employ a variety of psychological theories in the treatment of clients to achieve identified goals (Darnley-Smith & Patey 2003). Improvisation acts as a vehicle for communication within the therapeutic relationship and allows for the expression of emotions. The improvised music provides a connection to the unconscious of the client, providing information for learning, growth and the expression of self (Bruscia 2014; Darnley-Smith & Patey 2003).

The role of music in the clinical setting is to bolster balance and harmony within the mind, body and spirit of the individual (McCarthy 2016). Music therapy can be employed to provide education, identify strengths and personal values, and develop positive behavioral patterns. Reflection within music therapy upon problem solving skills, relationship skills and unconscious material that may drive pathological and destructive behavior has been shown to be effective with clients (McCarthy 2016). Music therapy has been found to assist in building neuroplasticity, enhancing cognitive functioning, reducing depressive and anxiety symptoms, and increasing wellbeing in clients (McCarthy 2016).

Drumming and shamanic trances

Rhythm and the vibration patterns of music have been shown to influence cognitive functioning, mood, affect and physiology, as well as brainwave functioning, as reflected in EEG scans (Sideroff & Angel 2013). Listening to music composed by Mozart resulted in a decrease in alpha and theta frequencies within the brain. The reduction of alpha and theta frequencies occurred most prominently in the left hemisphere of the brain and is indicative of an improvement in cognitive functioning of the individual (Sideroff & Angel 2013).

Shamanic drumming to achieve an altered state of consciousness (ASC) has been shown to involve a change in theta brainwaves (Flor-Henry et al. 2017; Maxfield 1990; Sideroff & Angel 2013). Drumming to attain an ASC consists of creating and holding a steady rhythm composed of 4–4½ drum beats per second for a duration of 13–15 minutes (Flor-Henry et al. 2017; Maxfield 1990; Sideroff & Angel 2013).

Within research studies, the result of holding this rhythm and beat was a reported increase in theta brainwaves of 4–8 cycles per second in the right hemisphere of the brain (Flor-Henry *et al.* 2017; Maxfield 1990). The increase in theta brainwaves in the right hemisphere is characteristic of entering into a temporary ASC (Maxfield 1990). An ASC involves experiencing a shift in a mental state of consciousness, along with any of the following sensations: visual imagery, creative flow or a loss of a sense of time, a sensation of flying, pressure on the body, a sense of a spiritual journey or visitation, along with a shift in a mental state of consciousness (Flor-Henry *et al.* 2017; Maxfield 1990). Shamanic trances are considered to be voluntary and self-induced. Shamanic ASCs hold a historical purpose of social unification and acted as an intervention for healing across a wide variety of tribal cultures and settings (Flor-Henry *et al.* 2017).

Sonic vibrations in conjunction with physical exertion and the release of emotions through drumming have been shown to be conducive to achieving an altered state of consciousness (Winkelman 2003). An altered state of consciousness achieved through drumming facilitates the ability to "synchronize the frontal lobes of the brain" through which there is a process of "integrating non-verbal information from the lower brain structures to the frontal cortex and producing insight" (Winkelman 2003). It is theorized that the integration process, along with drumming, acts to reduce and possibly remove the impact of traumatic experiences (Winkelman 2003).

Within the cultures of American Indians, the symbolic nature of the drum is sacred and is an essential component to rituals (Dickerson *et al.* 2014). The playing of the drum is a central feature in hunting ceremonies and in storytelling events. The drum is used to provide emphasis and acts to add cohesion between members of the community. The rhythms played on the drum are believed to assist and instill psychological, emotional and physical healing in individuals involved in the rituals and ceremonies (Dickerson *et al.* 2014).

Drum circles and music are used in therapeutic settings to "facilitate a sense of belonging, intimacy, togetherness and connectedness" (Bensimon *et al.* 2008). Within the group process of therapy, music making provides opportunities for assumption of social roles, expression of emotions, a sense of a purpose in life, a sense of belonging, emotional regulation and access to autobiographical and traumatic memories, as well as developing spiritual connections (Bensimon *et al.* 2008; Faulkner 2012; Longhofer & Floersch 1993; Mank 2019).

Musical improvisation within a therapeutic setting, utilizing psychodynamic theory along with emotional processing, has been shown to be effective in the treatment of depressive symptoms (Erkkilä *et al.* 2019). The nonverbal musical improvisation allows for manifestations of abstract and emotional content that lead to the access and processing of autobiographical memories, experiences, metaphor and images. The verbal processing of the emotional, visual and autobiographical content within the clinical group environment plays a key role in positive therapeutic outcomes (Erkkilä *et al.* 2019). The stages of therapy during musical improvisation within a therapeutic setting include: 1) arousal of emotional content; 2) acknowledgment of the emotions with emotional regulation; 3) processing of the emotions through the symbolic form of music and potentially creating meaning from the material brought up in the music making experience (Erkkilä *et al.* 2019). The making of music in a spontaneous and flexible manner that is based in creativity and within a reciprocal relationship, between a music therapist and a client, has been shown to be efficacious in numerous populations and settings (Tomaino 2014; Wigram 2004).

Creativity

There are three criteria that define whether an idea or product is considered creative (Kaufman & Sternberg 2007). First, an idea must be innovative and original. The second criterion stipulates that the original idea must hold potential for being useful or purposeful for a specific task. The third criterion is that the idea or product must be considered to be of high quality (Boccia *et al.* 2015; Kaufman & Sternberg 2007; Lhommée *et al.* 2014; Thagard & Stewart 2011). Previous research indicates that the highest predictor of creativity is originality, which influences the idea or product's ability to provide purpose and usefulness (Thomson & Jaque 2017). It is theorized that engagement in creativity through music stimulates the neural networks and subcortical regions of the brain, thereby reducing the activity of the lateral prefrontal cortex, and inhibits critical self-monitoring (Tomaino 2014). Simultaneously, there is activation in the medial prefrontal cortex, an area associated with self-expression and autobiographical memories.

Hinz (2009) postulated that creativity is a result of, and dependent upon, the development and maturation process that occurs in the prefrontal cortex of the human brain. Creativity has the potential to increase from childhood to adulthood. Because of the normal aging process, levels of creativity reduce—beginning around age 60—as a result of a decline in executive functioning (Hinz 2009). With the normal aging process, the brain experiences a loss of working memory and cognitive flexibility, limiting the ability to form novel and innovative connections and ideas (Hinz 2009). The somatic senses have the potential to stimulate cognition, thereby influencing behaviour, and are perceived to be the basis of emotion (Burns 1980; Hinz 2009). Neurological stimulation, provided by sensory information, may engage long-term memories and promote original and unusual connections within the brain (Hinz 2009).

Creativity acts as a mechanism for self-expression, regulates and contains thoughts and emotions, and provides opportunities for unique and original ideas, leading to self-understanding (Chapman 2014). Through the symbolic form of the expressive arts and the therapeutic relationship, the client can discover meaning. The therapist exercises skills and instincts to determine the appropriate approaches and directives within therapy. The art promotes opportunities for the creation of symbolic meaning independent of verbal language (Chapman 2014). The expressive arts provide a means for individuals to initiate social relationships and to experience membership of the community at large (Baumann 2007; Dixon 2007; Galligan 2000; Koc 2012; Paukert *et al.* 2010).

Improvisation

There are two forms of improvisation: clinical musical improvisation and musical improvisation (Gardstrom 2014). Clinical musical improvisation involves a music therapist and a client; original music is created, within the therapeutic relationship, with the goals of assessment and can also be used as a form of treatment (Gardstrom 2014). The client and the therapist use music to interact. The resulting music embodies a range of aesthetic properties and emotional expression that is reflective of the therapeutic relationship (Gardstrom 2014). Clinical improvisation involves the utilization of musical improvisation within a setting encompassing trust and emotional support in order to address the needs and goals of the client or clients (Wigram 2004). The music therapist draws upon theory, evidence-based practice and the predetermined goals or objectives identified by the client and therapist to guide the therapeutic use of improvisation (Gardstrom 2014).

Musical improvisation refers to musical opportunities and experiences between individuals that hold creative significance with the aim of producing music (Gardstrom 2014). There is no attempt or goal to develop therapeutic rapport or outcomes between the individuals creating music (Gardstrom 2014). Musical improvisation is defined as a sequence or combination of sounds that are created with a structure or framework that includes a beginning and an end (Wigram 2004).

Wigram (2004) describes musical improvisation as an uninhibited and changeable method of creating original music. Improvised music is a challenging way to create music and has the ability to increase anxiety levels within the individuals playing or singing the original music. It is up to the facilitator to create and nourish an environment that encourages an attitude of acceptance and enthusiasm for all that emerges in the experience (Wigram 2004). Music is a language in its own right; one with syntax and semantic components. Melody possesses many aspects of verbal language, including inflection and phrases that provide a base to evoke meaning within the musical improvisation. Improvised music is replete with the characteristics and emotions of the creator of the piece and conveys their affect, emotional content and values or attitudes (Wigram 2004).

Drum circles

Hull (2006) describes drum circles as a means to "build community with an intention to serve, to inspire and to reach beyond what separates us" (pp.22–23). Employing creativity to play improvised rhythms together, in a group environment, creates unity and connects one to one's own sense of humanity and community (Hull 2006). When the group synchronizes to a common pulse or rhythm, entrainment is achieved and hopefully maintained (Winkelman 2003). It is at the juncture of entrainment, via rhythm, that drum circle participants become engaged in the present moment and form a sense of connection that transcends the differences that separate one from another (Hull 2006). Hand percussion instruments are used to create improvised rhythmic experiences that beget unity, a sense of belonging and the expression of emotions (Hull 2006; Mank 2019).

Drum circles provide opportunities to learn through participation in an entertaining experience within a responsive environment (Knysh 2013). The safe and supportive environment of drum circles are founded upon "understanding, communication, respect, and celebration of similarities and differences" (Knysh 2013, p.1). Nonverbal communication within the musical improvisation of drumming bridges the barriers of language, thereby encouraging cross-cultural and global alliances among members of the group. The drum circle facilitator guides the members of the group, albeit strangers at the start, to locate the rhythmic pulse through which connection and community are formed (Knysh 2013). As the members of the drum circle find form within the entrainment of the pulse, communication and personal expression emerge while working toward the mutual goal of using creativity to make communal music (Knysh 2013, Mank 2019).

In order to achieve and maintain entrainment, collaboration and flexibility between all members of the drum circle are required (Knysh 2013). The drum or instrument selected to play assigns a role and voice to the person playing. The bass drum, often the largest diameter drum, helps anchor the pulse; the smaller drums provide a higher pitch that soars over the bass and can provide the melody (Mank 2019). The members of the drum circle must listen to the others and adapt their rhythms and playing styles to match the rest of the group or the rhythm will devolve into chaos (Knysh 2013). The collaboration between members of the group provides opportunities for members to take leadership roles, support fellow members, communicate nonverbally, build relationships, exercise creativity, express emotions and work as a team (Hull 2006; Knysh 2013; Mank 2019).

Stevens (2017) writes that drum circles call upon a primal urge to relate to, support and nonverbally communicate with others in an ancient and aesthetic form of beauty: namely music.

The drum becomes an instrument for social and musical engagement while providing time for self-reflection (Faulkner 2012). Faulkner (2012) conducted drum circles with Aboriginal youth who showed resistance to verbal therapy, and utilized a protocol called DRUMBEAT. The drum circles utilized the physical activity of drumming, which was conducted in a non-judgmental environment. The DRUMBEAT protocol of drumming with peers in a facilitated drum circle acted to provide safety, experiential learning, stimulated attention and concentration; it improved self-esteem, and increased a sense of belonging and connection to peers and community (Faulkner 2012). Participation in drum circles has been shown to provide relaxation and improve fine motor skills while providing physical activity (Bittman *et al.* 2001).

Bittman *et al.* (2001) conducted a research study with participants (described as normal) to determine whether drumming resulted in immune-enhancing effects for them. The study attempted to measure depressive symptoms, plasma cortisol, plasma dehydroepiandrosterone, plasma dehydroepiandrosterone-to-cortisol ratio, natural killer cell activity, lymphokine-activated killer cell activity, plasma interleukin-2, and plasma interferon-gamma. The results showed an increase in dehydroepiandrosterone-to-cortisol ratios, an increase in activity of the natural killer cells, and an increase in lymphokine-activated killer cells. There were no alterations in the plasma interleukin 2 or interferon gamma, nor were there any changes in depressive symptoms. The results indicate that drumming is an intervention that has the potential to regulate "neuroendocrine and neuroimmune parameters"—that is, in contradiction to the typical stress response (Bittman *et al.* 2001, p.38). These results suggest that drumming enhances the immune system of people who participate in drum circles. The nonjudgmental environment and group cohesion experienced from being in a drum circle lessened the normal stress response of the participants in this study (Bittman *et al.* 2001). This study suggests that group drumming may prove beneficial to individuals coping with chronic illness, although further long-term study is required (Bittman *et al.* 2001).

Drum circles can be facilitated or non-facilitated (the facilitator of a facilitated drum circle guides the members). The non-facilitated drum circle is focused on creating an improvised song with improvised rhythms (Cormier 2019). It is through listening to the rhythms created that one may be taken on a rhythmic or spiritual journey (Cormier 2019). The community drum circle is about bringing people together to form community, unity and peace while experiencing the joy of drumming (Cormier 2019).

The facilitator of a drum circle guides the members into a tempo that fits the skill level and abilities of the group (Hull 2006; Stevens

2017; Mank 2019). The goal is to find unity and entrainment while the group finds a sense of cohesion and belonging (Hull 2006; Stevens 2017; Mank 2019). The role of the facilitator is to address the needs of the group, which may include directives of sculpting, tempo or call and response without being a performer. The facilitator is in service to the group (Hull 2006; Stevens 2017; Mank 2019).

Conclusion

Music has been an integral part of the daily life and rituals of humans for centuries (Bittman *et al.* 2001; Cook & British Museum 2013). Improvisational drumming utilizes creativity and provides therapeutic benefits that include improved mood, a greater sense of belonging and a reduction in the normal stress response in humans (Bittman *et al.* 2001; Faulkner 2012). Within the development of identity and sense of self, music has figured prominently as the agent of change (DeNora 2000; Rolvsjord & Stige 2015). The values of a culture and community are reflected in music and have been shown to influence mood, spirituality, personality and memory of said community (DeNora 2000).

Music and drum circles offer opportunities to express emotions, build sociocultural identity and unite members of the community (Bensimon *et al.* 2008; Wanjala & Kebaya 2016). The creative use of music holds potential to stimulate areas of the brain that may help in achieving an ASC, connection to the collective unconscious and to previously unknown aspects of self (Jung 1963; Rugenstein 2000). Through music, music therapy and drum circles, therapeutic growth and change are possible. Drum circles based in creativity offer opportunities for stimulating neural networks of the brain, expressing emotions and instilling meaning (Tomaino 2014). Music offers developmental, emotional and spiritual growth that influences an individual's values and sense of self while offering a sense of belonging and community.

CHAPTER 5

Drum History and Drum Making

Drums come in a variety of sizes, shapes and styles that correlate to materials easily available to the region and culture that builds the drum (Waring 2007). The broad definition of what encompasses a drum includes one or more membranes stretched tightly over a chamber that has resonating properties (Dean 2012). The drum is then beaten with a body part, mallet or stick to produce a sound (Dean 2012). Historically, ancient flutes and rasps were made from bones. It is believed that many of those which exist today were created by Neanderthals and are tens of thousands of years old (Dean 2012; Waring 2007). Drums, on the other hand, were created from natural and impermanent materials such as wood and animal hide (Waring 2007), which means it may be impossible to know exactly when the first ones were made and played. Within the artwork that archeologists recovered from Mesopotamia, dating back to 3,000 B.C.E., there are images of drums, which suggests that drums existed and were played during that time period. There are statuettes that are believed to be dated to 2,000 B.C.E. from Babylonia of figures holding and playing frame drums (Waring 2007). Drums were a symbol of prominence and authority and can be found in nearly all cultures throughout time (Bensimon *et al.* 2008; Waring 2007).

Drumming and spirituality
The drum was considered to be a sacred instrument that could connect the player to the spiritual realm and the divine (Dissanayake 1995;

Murrell 2010; Waring 2007). Cultures that believe that living beings possess souls venerate the spirit within the natural products used to create the drum, thereby rendering it a spiritual and sacred object (Waring 2007). Music and drums were, and still are, used in ritual and spiritual practice to elevate the experience (Dissanayake 1995; Murrell 2010). The practitioners of the Santeria religion use drums and the triangle instrument to create an opening into, and experience a spiritual connection with, an alternative reality (Murrell 2010).

The drum is viewed as a sacred object within the American Indian culture (Dickerson *et al.* 2014). Within this culture, the drum acts to provide accentuation to storytelling and hunting ceremonies, as well as serving as a source of cohesion within the community. The rhythms played on the drum are thought to provide sacred medicine and healing on a physical, emotional and spiritual level (Dickerson *et al.* 2014). Drumming provides a method to cultivate a connection to a cultural identity and heritage, improve self-concept and increase self-esteem. Dickerson *et al.* (2014) conducted a study with drumming as a therapeutic intervention, whereby participants reported a reduction in substance abuse and improvement of mood.

Babtunde Olatunji was from Nigeria and is credited with bringing drum circles, the art of drumming and cultural awareness in regard to drumming and his experience of Nigeria to America (Hull 2006; Wolf 2016). By using voice and the drum as instruments, the spiritual world can be accessed and called into the present moment (Wolf 2016). It is also believed that through the use of the voice and drumming, the soul can be freed (Wolf 2016). The drum serves several additional purposes: It can be used as method of communication between people, at ceremonies as well as in battle (Bensimon *et al.* 2008; Wolf 2016). Within the context of social interaction, the drum can be used to synchronize repetitive actions such as catching nets, planting or harvesting crops. Drums can be used for healing while in an altered state of consciousness that allows for a broader and heightened sense of awareness, relaxation, attention and sense of presence (Wolf 2016).

Within the context of ritual, music initiates a sense of self-transcendence that is categorized as a detached aesthetic experience (Dissanayake 1995). During the detached aesthetic experience an individual may relinquish control and experience a sense of dissolution of boundaries and a sense of timelessness (Dissanayake 1995). Music and ritual have been used as a method to join with, and incorporate, the physical and spiritual realms and to access altered states of consciousness (Rugenstein 2000). The experience of connecting to something greater than self within an altered state of consciousness provides access to the unconscious, catharsis and greater insight (Rugenstein 2000).

Rhythm

Rhythm is vital to all humans—basic survival revolves around the rhythms of breath and the heartbeat (Friedman 2000). The first sound an infant hears within the womb is the mother's heartbeat. Friedman (2000) notes that "[i]nfants who receive steady, strong rhythmic messages through rocking with loving sounds from a caregiver, have quicker visual and auditory development" (p.24). Humans organize daily life and routine around the circadian rhythms of the wake/sleep cycle and physiology of the body, which includes hormones, saliva, body temperature and mood (Germain & Kupfer 2008). Vibrations from the playing of a drum have the ability to alter mood and shift perceptions (Friedman 2000). The patterning of sound through rhythm and repetition provides a sense of order and control while offering an opportunity for self-expression (Dissanayake 1995). Creating art, via rhythm, appears to be a trait in humans that contributes to positive feelings of mastery, reduction of anxiety, and a greater sense of security (Dissanayake 1995).

Gender and drumming

In the cave paintings from Mesopotamia dating back to the beginning of the 3rd century B.C.E., there is an image of a female holding a frame drum (Dean 2012). Women figured prominently in ancient pagan religions and worshiping, with the frame drum symbolizing the significance of goddesses (Dean 2012). This suggests that the male dominance of modern drumming was not the case in ancient times. With the rise of patriarchal rule and Christianity, the playing of music and drumming by women was disparaged as a way to reduce matriarchal reverence and worship (Dean 2012).

It should be noted that in modern times, the drum and drumming have been considered a masculine object and activity (Dean 2012).

This could be due to the drum's association with communication in war and battles (Dean 2012). The modern-day culture and perceived identity of drummers is predominately masculine (Smith 2013). In many American Indian tribes, women did not make or play the drums in public (Dickerson *et al.* 2012). In many tribes the women's role was to stand behind the male drummers and sing. A belief held by some American Indian tribes is that each gender has specific and unique powers. If a woman were to touch a drum, then the powers from both genders would mix, causing bad luck (Dickerson *et al.* 2012). In some American Indian tribes, women may play hand drums privately for the purpose of personal healing (Dickerson *et al.* 2012).

The Asabano tribe in Papua New Guinea had cultural norms that prohibited women and boys from playing the drum (Lohmann 2007). It was believed that the sound the drum produces is recognized as the sound that emerges from the vagina of a woman during intercourse. Therefore, the act of playing a drum is symbolic of the drummer having sexual relations with the women present during the musical event or ritual (Lohmann 2007). In regard to the symbolic meaning, it was considered inappropriate for boys before the ritual of initiation and education to even touch a drum (Lohmann 2007). Women were never allowed to touch or play a drum because of its symbolic nature and the cultural mores of the Asabano tribe (Lohmann 2007).

Drumming has many cultural and spiritual connotations. The social and cultural identity of drumming, rhythm and drummers may be shaped by the long history of the role of drumming in human civilization (Dean 2012; Dickerson *et al.* 2012; Lohmann 2007; Smith 2013). Understanding the cultural mores, standards and beliefs are important when assuming roles within a multicultural drum circle.

Personal drum making history

In determining a process by which to make a drum, it is important not to appropriate a drum from another culture. The tubano drum is a self-standing tubular drum with straight sides and a drumhead on one end that was created and manufactured by an American drum manufacturer, Remo. The use of this style of drum does not specifically appropriate another culture and allows for easy playing for children and adults. The drum can be played with mallets or by hand.

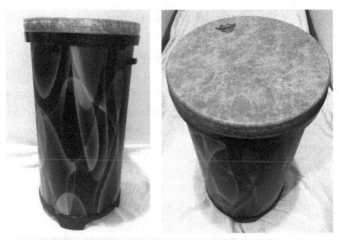

Figure 5.1: Tubano drum

I began making drums after being challenged by a music therapist to find a way to combine music therapy and art therapy. While contemplating the challenge, I was at a facility that sold donated items to avoid adding to landfills. I found a bin full of cast-off paper cores. Paper cores are tubes made of paper material and are thick-walled to support rolls of sheet paper, such as newsprint or butcher paper (similar to the cardboard tubes used for paper towels). The cores that I found had ⅜ inch walls and were 7 inches in diameter. The thick walls were strong enough to hold the paper cores' diameter and overall shape when the rawhide drumhead was attached and shrunk to fit the tube. The paper cores did make an adequate drum. However, given their small diameter, it was hard to play the drum with the hands because of the limited space on the drumhead. In addition, the length of the drum was too short to play as a self-standing drum while sitting in a chair.

I wanted to have larger-diameter drums that produced deeper tones and that could self-stand, so I began to look at different sizes and types of tubes. The tubes used to pour cement footings come in different diameters and can be cut to size (that is, in order to be able to play the drums while sitting in a chair). I recommend using tubes that are at least 10 inches in diameter. Within a moderate-size drum circle, a 14 inch diameter drum will act as a bass drum while still being relatively easy to make and transport. For this reason, I usually make three sizes of drums: 10, 12 and 14 inches in diameter. The tubes have a much thinner wall thickness than the paper cores and do need to be modified so that when the wet hide is attached and shrunk to fit, the walls do not cave in toward the center.

HOW TO MAKE A TUBANO DRUM

What you need

Before starting any project, proper safety equipment should be used and all tools should be handled with care and operated with caution, following all safety guidelines.

Equipment

- Safety glasses
- Snug-fitting work gloves (optional)
- Handsaw
- Sandpaper (medium and fine grit)
- Clamps (at least 6, with more required for tubes with larger diameters or if gluing both ends of the tube at once)
- Paintbrushes
- Marker pen or pencil
- Scissors
- Sheet of thick paper or cardstock (A3 size) for the drumhead template
- Piece of string
- Hole punch
- Leather-cutting scissors
- Awl
- Hammer
- Miter box
- Power drill
- Nail set tool
- Phillips head screwdriver
- Masking tape

Materials

- 1 long cement footing tube (22 inches long with a diameter of at least 10 inches)

- 2 short cement footing tubes (4 inches long with a diameter of at least 10 inches)
- Wood glue
- Gesso
- Acrylic paint
- Camper seal foam tape ($\frac{3}{16}$ inches thick x $1\frac{1}{4}$ inches wide; normally sold in lengths of 30 ft)
- Cow rawhide (wide enough to cut a circle 3 inches wider in diameter than the cement footing tube)
- Upholstery tacks (normally sold in packs of 100)
- Piece of pine wood ($\frac{3}{4}$ inch wide x $\frac{3}{4}$ inch thick x 36 inches long)
- Piece of pine wood ($\frac{3}{4}$ inch wide x $\frac{1}{4}$ inch thick x 6 inches long, or if that is not available, a piece of pine wood $\frac{3}{4}$ inch wide x $\frac{1}{8}$ inch thick x 6 inches long will work but needs to be double the length, or 12 inches long)
- 4 long finish nails (4D $1\frac{1}{2}$ inches long)
- Wood putty
- Liquid acrylic paint in a variety of colors
- Wood stain
- Polyurethane or lacquer
- 8 pan head chrome self-drilling screws (No. 8 diameter x $1\frac{1}{2}$ inches long)
- 4 furniture glides, supplied with 4 screws

Method
Fabrication using tubes
STEP 1: TUBE SELECTION AND MODIFICATION

Cement footing tubes can be purchased at most hardware stores and can be cut with a power or hand saw. Each drum requires a total of 30 inches in length from the same-size diameter tube (in three different pieces). Care should be taken when cutting tubes to ensure a 90-degree (perpendicular) cut to the wall. It is important to have a smooth and level surface to ensure a level drum and a unified sound from the drumhead. If cutting the drum yourself, make sure you place the tubes on a level surface to prevent injury, and follow the manufacturer's instructions for the cutting tool you are using. I recommend paying to have the tubes cut to size by a power saw if the hardware store offers that option. Feet will need to be attached to lift the tubing off the floor to allow the sound, or vibration, to escape from the bottom. The total length of the drum will be 25 inches after attaching the wooden feet and furniture glides.

Cut the long tube so that it is 22 inches in length. Two sections of tube (4 inches long and of the same diameter as the 22 inches tube) also need to be cut in order to reinforce the top and bottom of the long tube. The 4 inch long sections then need to be made smaller to fit inside the long tube. To do this, make two vertical cuts approximately ½ inch away from each other along the length of both of the 4 inch tubes—in other words, remove a vertical ½ inch section (see Figure 5.2).

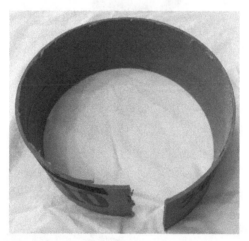

Figure 5.2: Modified reinforcement tube

Sand both ends of the inner wall of the long tube from the outer edges for 4 inches in length to allow for better adhesion of the glue used to bond the long and short tubes together. Apply wood glue to the outer surface of the 4 inch long tubes before inserting them inside the 22 inch tube, lining up the edges to ensure a level, perpendicular surface to the walls of the tube. Position clamps to hold the 4 inch long rings in place inside the 22 inch long tube until the glue is dry (see Figure 5.3). If the drum can be placed horizontally to dry, then both ends of the long tube can be reinforced at the same time. If the tube needs to stand upright (because of space restrictions or a limited number of clamps), then only one end should be glued at a time. It is recommended that the tubes be allowed to dry for approximately 24 hours. It is important that the vertically cut edges of the inner tubes do not meet inside the long tube. When the upholstery tacks are hammered into the outer tube and into the inner tube, the force of the nails can separate the two tubes if the inner tube does not have extra space between its vertical edges. Once the glue has dried, remove the clamps and inspect the edges of the tube. If the edges are not smooth, use medium grit sandpaper to sand them to ensure the surface is level, perpendicular to the walls and smooth (see Figure 5.4).

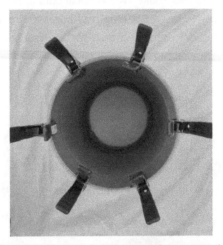

Figure 5.3: Gluing and clamping reinforcement tube

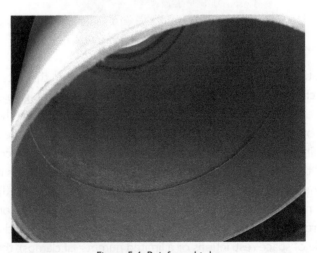

Figure 5.4: Reinforced tube

STEP 2: PREPARING THE OUTER WALL OF THE DRUM

Paint the outer tube with gesso and allow it to dry. The top and bottom edges of the tube should also be painted with gesso to seal the tube. When the first coat is dry, apply another coat of gesso. I prefer to apply the second coat to the surface in the opposite direction to the first coat to reduce the chance of drips or missing spots on the tube. Once the second coat is dry, I apply a third coat of gesso in the same direction as the first coat. This means that if I use vertical strokes for the first coat, I use horizontal strokes for the second coat, and vertical strokes for the third coat.

Once the gesso is dry, the outside of the tube can be decorated with acrylic paint. Mank (2019) found that after developing a sense of belonging between members of the drumming group after ten weeks of drumming, participants created a symbol of self on the drum in a convivial manner during the group art sessions. Participants who created the symbol of self on the drum prior to the start of the ten-week drumming sessions did not experience as rich an atmosphere where mastery was celebrated and the sense of creativity increased due to the artistic rendering. For this reason, it is recommended to wait to paint the symbol of self on the drum until after the participants of the therapeutic drum circle have played together and formed a cohesive group (Mank 2019). The tube can be painted with a base coat of acrylic paint if desired. The drumhead can be attached to the tube and the symbol can be painted or attached at a later date. However, if the drum is not created within a therapeutic group environment, then it can be painted with a symbol of self before attaching the drumhead.

STEP 3: APPLYING CAMPER SEAL TAPE

When the outside of the drum is complete and the gesso or the acrylic paint is dry, apply the camper foam to the inside of the drum. Measure approximately ⅝ inch down from what will be the top of the drum on the inside of the tube and make a mark with a marker pen or pencil. Do this about every 2 inches around the circumference of the inside of the drum. Take the camper seal foam and place the adhesive side against the inside of the drum, making sure to line up the long edge of the foam with the marks you have previously made. Working around the circumference of the inside of the drum, carefully press the foam onto the tube's surface to ensure there are no air bubbles and the foam is adhering. Cut the foam with scissors once it meets the beginning of the foam strip attached to the tube so that it forms a complete circle inside the tube. Now add another layer of foam on top of the first. It is recommended that the second layer's start/end point is offset by a few inches from the first, although the top and bottom sides should be aligned. (If the start/end seams are the same on both layers, there is a chance the foam tape might peel up.) The purpose of applying foam to the inside of the tube is to encase the upholstery tacks and provide some safety if one were to reach inside the drum (see Figure 5.5).

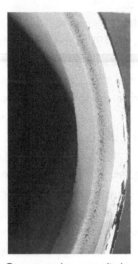

Figure 5.5: Camper seal tape applied to inner wall

Making the drumhead

Rawhide is generally used as the drumhead for this type of drum. Plastic sheets or fabric could be used, but they tend to be more temporary. I often work with elders who are in the Integrity versus Despair stage of development (Erikson 1963). During this period, the elder is coping with the realization that there is a finite amount of time left in this life, so creating a legacy and finding meaning are important aspects to consider. I wanted to create a drum that has longevity in sound and aesthetics to ensure that the elder could use the drum as a legacy object. Therefore, I recommend the use of rawhide as the drumhead because of its more lasting qualities as well as its aesthetically pleasing visual and acoustic features.

STEP 1: MAKING A TEMPLATE

Creating a template for cutting the rawhide helps with the cutting of round circles and for placement of the upholstery tacks on the rawhide. Begin by getting a piece of thick paper such as cardstock or Bristol board. Draw a circle on the paper 3 inches larger in diameter than the tube's diameter (for example, if you are using a 10 inches diameter tube, then draw a 13 inches diameter circle). If you don't have an object with a circle of the appropriate size to trace, make a centerpoint mark on the paper. Draw a vertical line that is longer than the diameter of the drumhead through the centerline on the paper. Draw a horizontal line through the centerpoint that is longer than the diameter of the drumhead, so that there is a cross on the paper. It is helpful to have the lines perpendicular to one another. This can be done by measuring from side to side of the paper to create a straight line or by using a T-square as shown in Figure 5.6.

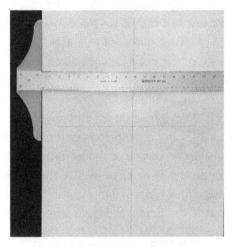

Figure 5.6: Centerlines of template

Now take a piece of string that is several inches longer than the required radius for the circumference of the tube and tie a pencil to it. Hold the pencil upright and measure a radius that is 1½ inches more than the radius of the tube. Holding the string in place on the centerpoint drawn on the paper, draw a circle. Reduce the length of the string by ¾ of an inch and draw another circle on the paper inside the first. Finally, reduce the length of the string by ¾ of an inch and draw another circle that has the same circumference as the tube (see Figure 5.7).

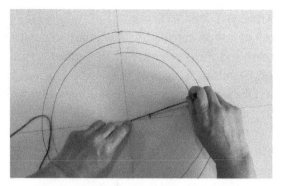

Figure 5.7: Drawing diameters on template

Take a ruler, that is 3 inches longer than the diameter of the drum, and measure 1 inch from the intersection of the centerline on the paper and the drawn middle circle. Make a mark on the middle circle. Position the ruler so that it aligns with the mark, the center point of all the circles and extends to the opposite side of the middle circle. Draw a short line on the mark and repeat on the opposite side of the middle circle. Continue to measure, make marks and draw short lines until the entire circumference of the circle is divided into 1 inch sections. These marks will be the centerpoint of the hole punches to mark where the upholstery tacks will be hammered on the tube. Cut the paper along the outer circle line. Take a hole punch and punch out holes using the marks on the middle circle as centerpoints for the hole punch. Make four more holes, with an awl or a similar type of instrument, on a protected surface, on the inner circle where the centerlines intersect with the circle. These four holes will mark where to place the wooden feet on the bottom of the tube (see Figure 5.8).

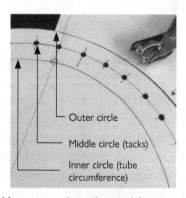

Outer circle

Middle circle (tacks)

Inner circle (tube circumference)

Figure 5.8: Measuring and punching tack location on template

STEP 2: PREPARING THE RAWHIDE

Rawhide can be purchased from leather companies locally or online. Cow rawhide works well and is less expensive than more exotic animal hides. The amount of rawhide depends on the size and number of drums being made. Rawhide normally has one side that is smoother than the other. The side that is smoother, more even and seems to have a grain is the outside of the hide and will be the outside of the drumhead. Make sure to use a section of rawhide that does not have holes (and ideally no brand marks), and that is of even thickness to ensure ease in stretching and uniformity of tones.

Take the template and place it on the outside of the rawhide. While holding the template in place, use a pencil to trace the outer circle of the template onto the rawhide. Then mark each of the hole punches from the middle circle onto the rawhide (see Figure 5.9).

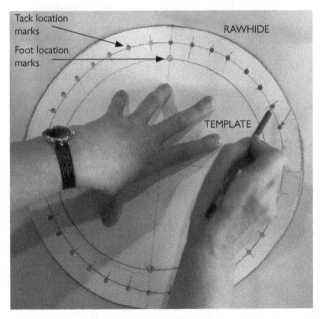

Figure 5.9: Using template to mark rawhide

The rawhide is too stiff to cut in its dried state and therefore must be soaked overnight. Fill a bathtub or a children's plastic pool with enough water to cover the rawhide. Place it in the water and weigh it down with something waterproof and heavy to keep it submerged overnight. I use clean rocks or ceramic tiles.

STEP 3: ATTACHING THE RAWHIDE TO THE TUBE

Once the rawhide is saturated with water and is pliable, take it out of the water and cut along the outer circle drawn on the hide. When working with the wet hide, work quickly and keep out of the sun on a hot day as the hide may dry out while working with it, resulting in a less than pleasing tone from the drumhead. Center the rawhide circle on the opening of the tube that will be the top (see Figure 5.10).

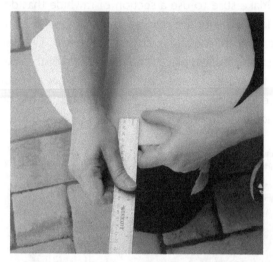

Figure 5.10: Centering prepared rawhide on tube

Take an awl and place it on the mark for the upholstery tack drawn on the rawhide. Using a hammer, push the awl through the rawhide and slightly into the tube, making a partial pilot hole for the upholstery tack. Remove the awl and place an upholstery tack through the rawhide and into the pilot hole on the tube. Hammer the tack into the tube. Rotate the tube 180 degrees. If the tube were a clock, the first tack would be hammered into the 12 o'clock position, and the second tack would be hammered into the 6 o'clock position.

Pull the hide so that it is taut and use the awl to make a hole through the hide and into the tube opposite the first hole. Again, place an upholstery tack into the hole and hammer into place, keeping the ide taut. Turn the tube 90 degrees and repeat the process. Turn the tube 180 degrees and repeat the process. Turn the tube 45 degrees and continue the stretching and nailing. Keep moving the drum and tacking the hide, making sure to alternate between the sides of the tube opening. The goal is to evenly attach the rawhide to the tube by rotating the tube and dividing the space until the circumference of the drum is covered with upholstery tacks spaced approximately 1 inch apart from one another and the hide is tightly stretched at the end of the tube (see Figure 5.11). Each piece of rawhide is unique and stretches differently, providing a different tone and aesthetic.

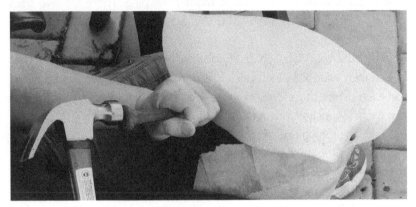

Figure 5.11: Attaching rawhide to tube

Let the hide and tube dry, hide side up, for several days until completely dry. The hide should have shrunk and the drum should produce three different tones when hit with the hand or mallet in different locations of the drumhead.

Making the feet for the drum

While the drum is drying, the feet can be made. Four feet provide stability. If weight is not a concern, mahogany makes a beautiful addition to the drum. If weight is an issue, pine or poplar wood make lightweight feet. The softer the wood, the more likely it will get scuffed and dented in transport. Pine and poplar are relatively inexpensive and can be replaced if necessary.

You can use a router to cut a vertical slot, approximately 2 inches deep, on the wooden foot. The drum, or tube wall, will be inserted into the slot. The slot and length of the foot should allow for at least 1 inch clearance between the bottom edge of the tube and the floor to allow the sound vibration to escape the tube. Not everyone has access to, or is comfortable using, a router. Therefore, the following instructions will be for constructing a foot with a handsaw, miter box and drill. There are risks in working with wood, and proper care is required. Please follow all safety instructions provided with the machines and materials used in this process.

STEP 1: MEASURING AND CUTTING THE WOOD

The feet in this instruction will be made from pine. There are two sizes of wood required for each foot; the outer parts are longer and the shim is shorter.

The outer part of each drum foot requires two pieces of wood that are ¾ inch wide x ¾ inch thick x 3¾ inches long. There are four feet for each drum; therefore, you will need eight pieces of cut wood that are each 3¾ inches in length.

Take the long piece of pine that is ¾ inch wide x ¾ inch thick x 36 inches long. Measure 3¾ inches from the end of the wood and make a pencil mark. Measure another 3¾ inches from that point and make another mark on the wood. Continue until all eight pieces are measured. Put the piece of wood in the miter box. Move the wood so that the mark lines up with the perpendicular line and is snug against the side of the miter box. Keep your fingers and hands away from the cutting edge of the saw while holding the wood tightly against the side of the miter box. Using a handsaw, cut through the wood. Repeat the process for each measured section of wood until you have eight pieces (see Figure 5.12).

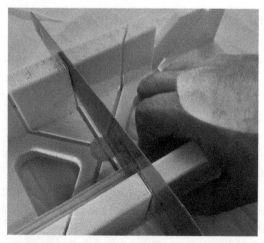

Figure 5.12: Cutting outer wood for drum feet

STEP 2: MEASURING, CUTTING AND GLUING THE SHIM

Select another piece of wood that is ¾ inch wide and ¼ inch thick, to match the width of the long pieces. If a piece of wood that is ¾ inch wide is unavailable, you can saw a wider piece to the appropriate width. This smaller piece of ¼ inch thick wood matches the thickness of the modified wall at the bottom of the tube and acts as a shim, or spacer, making a slot for the drum to slip into between the two longer pieces of wood. If ¼ inch thick wood is unavailable, glue two pieces of ⅛ inch thick wood together.

Assuming a ¼ inch thick piece of wood is unavailable, cut an ⅛ inch thick piece of wood to 1½ inches in length, while adhering to safety precautions. Cut two pieces of wood for each foot (i.e., eight pieces of ⅛ inch thick x 1½ inches long wood are needed per drum). Spread glue on the ¾ inch wide side of one piece of the ⅛ inch x 1½ inches cut wood and press a second piece of wood onto it, matching the ¾ inch wide x 1½ inches long sides together and making sure the edges are exactly aligned on all sides. Clamp the pieces together to ensure strong adhesion and allow 24 hours for drying prior to construction of the foot. Remove the clamp when the glue is dry and set (see Figure 5.13).

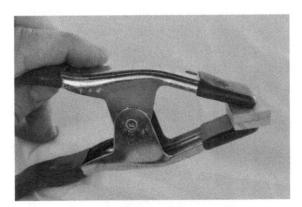

Figure 5.13: Gluing and clamping shim

STEP 3: GLUING THE SEPARATE PIECES OF WOOD TOGETHER

Glue the shim between both pieces of ¾ inch wide x ¾ inch thick x 3¾ inches long wood, making sure it is exactly aligned. Clamp, and allow the glue to dry for 24 hours. When the glue is dry, remove the clamps. The pieces of wood should be exactly aligned and solid on one end, with a slot that is ¼ inch across and 2¼ inches long on the other end (see Figure 5.14).

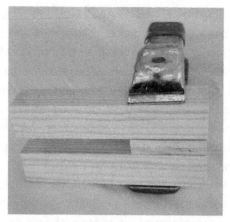

Figure 5.14: Gluing shim and outer wood together

STEP 4: ADDING AN ANGLE TO THE FOOT

To avoid the foot from becoming chipped or hurting someone, an angle can be created on one of the wood pieces of the foot at the end with the slot. Place the foot in the miter box. Using another piece of wood as a jig, align the foot with the 45-degree angle cut. Use tape with strong adhesive or a clamp to secure the wood acting as a jig to the miter box. This step is to keep the foot from slipping by securing the jig prior to cutting the angle. Make sure the wood is securely against the wall of the box and is held tightly, with all hands and fingers removed from the area. Saw the wood to remove the 90-degree angle and create a 45-degree angle (see Figure 5.15).

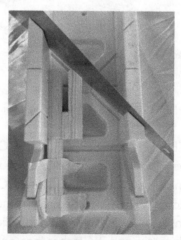

Figure 5.15: Cutting angle on wooden foot

STEP 5: SECURING THE WOOD

To ensure that the wooden foot is held tightly together, hammer a nail into the glued and solid section of the foot to secure all pieces of wood together. Since the side with the angle cut will go on the outside of the tube, the nail should be put in the solid section on the opposite side of the foot. In other words, the foot is positioned with the angle side downward while the nail is being hammered into place; that way, should the nail be visible, it will be toward the inside of the tube. Using a 4D x 1½ inches long finish nail, hammer it into the solid section of the wooden foot. Using the nail setting tool, hammer the head of the nail so that it is no longer exposed (see Figure 5.16). Fill the hole with wood putty and allow to dry.

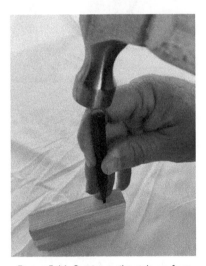

Figure 5.16: Setting nail on drum foot

STEP 6: FINISHING THE FOOT

The wooden foot should be sanded with 200 grit sand paper, after which it can be finished according to personal and aesthetic preference: painted with gesso and then, when dry, painted with acrylic paint; kept natural; or stained and wiped or sprayed with several coats of polyurethane, as directed by the manufacturer.

STEP 7: ATTACHING THE FOOT TO THE DRUM

Two pilot holes should be drilled into the wood on the part that has the opening and is not cut on an angle. Measure ¾ inch down from the top and make a mark in the center. Measure 1½ inches down from the top and make another mark. Take the drill and attach a 7/64 drill bit to it. Secure the wood mark side up on the flat surface. Drill two pilot holes through the first piece of wood and slightly into the other piece of wood on the end with the slot (see Figure 5.17). Use a pan head screwdriver, or pan head bit on the drill, to screw the No. 8 diameter 8 x 1½ inches long screws through the non-angled piece of wood and only slightly into the slot of the foot.

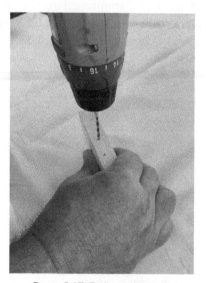

Figure 5.17: Drilling pilot holes

Turn the drum so that the end of the drum that will be the bottom is facing upward. Put the drum on a flat surface and place the template on the bottom of the tube. Mark the bottom with a pencil in the four holes made in the smallest diameter circle drawn. Take the foot and slide the end with the opening onto the wall of the drum with the angled side facing outward. The side with the two pilot holes should be facing toward the inside of the drum. Center the foot on the mark previously made. Do the same to the rest of the feet. Make sure they are centered, leveled and not at an angle.

Finish screwing the two No. 8 diameter x 1½ inches long screws through the wooden piece on the inside of the tube, the drum wall and into the back piece of the wooden foot (see Figure 5.18). Repeat for the other three feet .

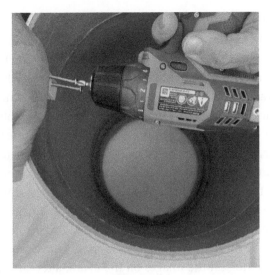

Figure 5.18: Attaching drum foot to tube

STEP 8: ATTACHING THE GLIDE TO THE WOODEN FOOT

Once the foot is attached to the drum, attach a 1 inch diameter rubber furniture pad (furniture glide) to the bottom of each wooden foot with the screw provided. Drill a pilot hole and then screw the glide into place with a screwdriver or drill (see Figure 5.19). It is important to have a rubber furniture pad on the drum to reduce additional vibration and provide a cleaner sound from the drum .

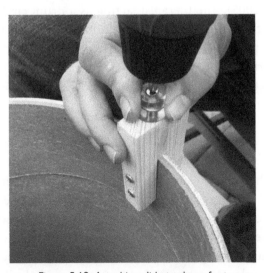

Figure 5.19: Attaching glide to drum foot

Creating the symbol of self

Within the therapeutic experience of art therapy and the drum circle, a symbol of self is suggested as the directive used to create the art on the drum. With the facilitation of an art therapist, the drum can become a transitional object for the owner of the drum and be part of a therapeutic experience within the drum circle (Winnicott 2005). The drum owner can complete a symbol from imagination, use templates to paint images, or use stickers or collage materials to complete the symbol of self on the drum. It is recommended that the drum owner uses acrylic paint on the tube/drum since it dries quickly and is waterproof. If using collage, care must be taken to completely coat the image with sealant so that the edges adhere tightly to the tube in order to avoid tears to the image while the drum is being transported. I have successfully used Modge Podge® to seal the images on the drum; alternatively, I make a solution of approximately one part water to two parts water-based glue.

The art therapist can work as the owner's third hand and assist the drum owner in creating an image that is reflective of what the individual feels represents their self (Kramer 1972). When the drum is complete, it can be used in the drum circle as a form of sublimation that redirects emotions in a socially acceptable manner which provides a sense of release (Kramer 1972). Playing a drum that acts as a transitional object within the safe environment of a therapeutic drum circle provides a way to express inner feelings and to explore new ways of being in the world (Winnicott 2005). The therapist, acting as a drum circle facilitator, along with the group members can utilize mirroring, modeling of socially acceptable behavior and positive regard for the participant to build rapport, attachment, transitional space and a sense of belonging, and assist in therapeutic growth and change (Kossak 2015; Mank 2019; Rogers 2007; Winnicott 2005).

Symbol of self and the ETC

Under the therapeutic care of an art therapist, a client can experience growth and change. The art therapist can utilize the ETC as an assessment tool or as a means to conceptualize materials and methods to best serve the client (Hinz 2009). Depending on the selection and use of materials, the art therapist may determine information processing of the client and develop a treatment plan to aid the removal of impediments to the client's processing. With therapeutic intervention, the movement from one level of the ETC to another should be gradual, especially if there is a perceived blockage in visual processing within the brain (Hinz 2009). Therapeutic interventions need to be conducted in such a manner that they address individual needs and do not overwhelm the client. The goal is for functioning at a Creative level (Hinz 2009). Effective information processing holds the potential to incorporate the functioning at all components and levels in order to achieve optimal visual processing of information on the Creative level (Hinz 2009).

KINESTHETIC COMPONENT

The creation of a symbol of self on the drum allows the art therapist to evaluate the visual processing of the participant. As stated earlier, the Kinesthetic/Sensory level is the least complex level of processing (Hinz 2009). The expressive arts that accentuate the Kinesthetic component include rhythm, movement and the discharge of energy. The Kinesthetic component is exemplified by arousal levels within the client. These can be at either extreme: increased and high energy; or low energy and lack of arousal (Lusebrink 2016). If the participant is creating a symbol of self and is painting the drum without regard to boundaries and is exhibiting either a great deal of energy or a diminished level of arousal and energy, then they may be functioning at the Kinesthetic component of the ETC (Hinz 2009; Lusebrink 2016). If there appears to be a blockage of visual processing in the participant, the art therapist could encourage the participant to focus on the sensory aspects of the mediums to move toward the Creative transition area of the Kinesthetic/Sensory level. The art therapist could also attempt to encourage the participant to identify boundaries or forms in an effort to move to the Perceptual/Affective level of the ETC.

SENSORY COMPONENT

The Sensory component of the ETC includes slow movements and an attention to the visual or tactile aspects of the art materials (Hinz 2009; Lusebrink 2016). The participant may be highly sensitive, both internally and externally, to the sensory-based stimuli of the art making process involved in creating a symbol of self on the drum (Hinz 2009). When creating a symbol of self, the participant may be focused on the colors or their ability to move and spread paint. Form and structure are not of great importance whereas the sensory aspects of the art materials are of significance (Hinz 2009).

The art therapist could draw the participant's attention to how the sensory stimuli affect the participant emotionally. The art therapist may offer the participant vibrant and rich hues of color with which to experiment. The rich hues and vibrant colors may stimulate emotions and help to move the participant to the Affective component and allow for processing of emotional experiences and memories (Hinz 2009).

PERCEPTUAL COMPONENT

The Perceptual component of the ETC can be recognized in the directive to make a symbol representing oneself on the drum through an increased ability to create formal elements within the artistic visual expression by means of line, shape and color (Hinz 2009). The definition and differentiation of figures and ground exemplify the Perceptual component. As with the other levels of the ETC, there can be divergent forms of expression. On the Perceptual component there can be defined boundaries and forms or a lack of forms and definition (Hinz 2009).

The art therapist could work with the participant to identify cognitive processes and to attempt to conceptualize and verbalize aspects of the symbol. The formation and identification of spatial elements in the symbol of self are aspects of the Cognitive component functioning (Hinz 2009).

AFFECTIVE COMPONENT

The Affective component of the ETC involves identification and expression of emotions or affect (Hinz 2009). Within the creation of art, there can be an emphasis upon intense hue or value displayed in the art materials. The opposite effect of functioning on the Affective component can be the use of color that is inappropriate for the subject matter of the image. There can be a lack of ability to distinguish figure from ground within the art image. Within the creation of a symbol of self, the art therapist should be attuned to the participant's use of art materials, their ability to distinguish form and boundaries, and the use of color and hue to express emotions (Hinz 2009). There could be an expression of symbolic meaning within the image created that could indicate possible movement toward the next and higher level containing the Symbolic component (Hinz 2009; Lusebrink 2016).

COGNITIVE COMPONENT

The Cognitive component involves the synthesis of line and shape that culminates in the formation of concepts and ideas, perception of spatial elements, and the ability to include printed words within the art (Hinz 2009; Lusebrink 2016). The art therapist should be aware of increased cognitive processing within the participant as a result of the art making of a symbol of self (Hinz 2009; Lusebrink 2016).

SYMBOLIC COMPONENT

The art images are evocative of emotion and symbolic meaning when the participant is functioning on the Symbolic component. The inverse aspects of the Symbolic component include the reversal of figure and ground as well the inclusion of aberrant and peculiar symbols (Lusebrink 2016). When operating at the Creative transition area, there are increased aspects of spirituality, discovery of unknown aspects of self and increased imagination (Hinz 2009; Lusebrink 2016).

Conceptualization of the expressive art processes through the theoretical and hierarchical framework of the ETC allows the art therapist to identify strengths and develop art interventions to remove visual information processing blockages in order to achieve integrated brain processing of the participant (Hinz 2009; Lusebrink 1991, 2010, 2016). The initiation point of the ETC is determined by the participant's selection and use of art materials. The movement from the initiation point of the ETC should be gradual in order to prevent the participant from becoming overwhelmed (Hinz 2009).

The creation of a symbol of self within the therapeutic milieu holds potential for the participant to explore life experiences and emotions with objectivity and creativity (Hinz 2009; Lusebrink 1991, 2010, 2016; Schaverien 1992). Operating with an integrated and creative manner holds potential to reduce depressive symptoms, hold intense emotions and improve self-esteem through the creative and symbolic process of art making (Jung 1963; Hinz 2009; Lusebrink 1991, 2020, 2016).

Conclusion

Drums and music are integral components of nearly all cultures on Earth. Drumming holds the potential to elevate a ceremony or ritual to something greater (Dissanayake 1995; Waring 2007). The music and the drumming experience have the potential for creating a sense of self-transcendence (Dissanayake 1995). The drum was considered sacred and acted as a means for spiritual connection (Dissanayake 1995; Murrell 2010; Waring 2007).

Traditionally, drums are made from the materials that are available and distinct to the cultures that create the drum (Waring 2007). This chapter detailed the multiple steps required for creating a drum that is self-standing and holds potential for becoming a legacy object depicting a symbol of self. Through the creation of a symbol of self, the art therapist can gain awareness of the visual processing of the participant and utilize art materials to initiate movement along the levels and poles of the ETC in order to enable creative functioning and integrated cognitive processing (Hinz 2009; Lusebrink 2010, 2016).

CHAPTER 6

Leading a Drum Circle

Drum circles comprise a domain where music and creativity are used as a form of self-expression within a group setting (Ratigan 2009). Drum circles act to unite the participants, transforming individual voices into a pronouncement of community through the efforts of the group (Ratigan 2009). Rhythm is a common denominator in the daily life of humans that connects us to oneself and to the universe. Humans are grounded in the rhythm of the heartbeat and breath along with the rhythm of the sun rising and setting and extending outward to include the revolutions and rhythms that exist in the universe (Ratigan 2009). Drumming provides an opportunity to ground oneself in rhythm while making connections to others and working toward a common goal of creating community (Hull 2006; Ratigan 2009). In nearly all cultures, throughout history, drumming and drum circles have brought people together to communicate, celebrate, make special, mourn and unite in a way that is no longer a universal process in modern-day life (Bensimon *et al.* 2008; Dissanayake 1995; Donovan 2015).

Structure of a drum circle

Each drum circle is unique to the time, place and individuals present. There is no specific recipe to follow within a therapeutic milieu in order to achieve growth and healing in the expressive arts of drumming, singing, movement and art therapy. Below is an outline of a general structure that assists in facilitating the experience for the group that can be modified as needed. Flexibility, recognition of the needs of the group, empathy for the participants and gratitude for their efforts are guiding principles that should be exercised by the facilitator in order to best serve the group.

1. Room selection

2. Circle set up

3. Welcoming and drum selection

    a. Experimentation

    b. Improvisation without facilitation

4. Introduction of facilitator

    a. Determine need for setting an intention

    b. Stretching and warm up

5. Meditation/becoming present

6. Facilitation

    a. Ice breaker exercise of names or songs as check-in

    b. Group improvisation and directives

7. Break

    a. Feedback

    b. Return to drumming

8. Facilitation

    a. Directives based on feedback

    b. Directives based on assessment and attunement

9. Check-out

    a. Feedback and check-out

    b. Stretch hands

10. Closing

    a. Thank the participants for coming

    b. Remind participants of next drum circle

    c. Dismantle the drum circle

Drum circle facilitation
Room selection and set up

The first step in leading a therapeutic drum circle is to select a room for the drum circle. It must have multiple exits and be located far enough away from other offices and rooms so as not to cause a disruption to the daily lives and activities of others. The room should also have a door that can be closed in order to help prevent the sound from disturbing others. Someone coming into the room and complaining about the "noise" will reduce the safety of the environment, negatively affect attunement and may adversely affect the cohesiveness of the group.

Tables and furniture should be moved to the edges of the room and the chairs should be arranged in a circle, leaving plenty of elbow room between the chairs. There should be at least two entrances into the circle that are wide enough for wheelchairs to move freely. Larger drum circles will need more entrances. Depending on the number of participants expected and the size of the room, concentric circles of chairs may be necessary. Spaces should be left in each circle of chairs to accommodate wheelchairs.

The space within the circle should be wide enough for the facilitator to move freely and for participants to enter and dance if desired (Ratigan 2009). The center space of the circle is often considered to be the orchestration spot (Hull 2006). The facilitator within the center space of the circle will provide direction and information and draw the attention of the group (Hull 2006).

The vibrations of the drums are quite powerful within the center space of the drum circle. For that reason, I often place a chair in the center of the space inside the circle for people to sit and feel the vibrations and rhythms of the drums. It is preferable for people who are having the space to experience the drumming experience, but who are not facilitating the drum circle or dancing, to be seated in order to not to distract the other members of the group.

Instrument selection and placement

The instruments selected for a drum circle should include a variety of hand percussion instruments. Shakers and rattles, bells and chimes, clave and rhythm sticks, or boom whackers provide a rich and interesting sound and rhythmic ingredient to the improvisational songs created in the drum circle. There is no limit to the variety of hand percussion instruments that can be selected. In a large circle where there are not enough drums, the drums and hand percussion instruments can be equally distributed around the circle to ensure everyone is provided with an instrument. At several points during the therapeutic drum circle, the participants can be asked to pass the instrument they are playing to the person on their right. This way, everyone gets to play a variety of instruments and their hands also get a rest from drumming.

If using handmade tubano drums, a variety of different diameter drums should be selected and evenly spaced around the circle. If using commercially purchased drums, try to get a variety of styles with two of each kind so that the style of instrument is evenly distributed around the circle and more than one person has a chance to play that particular style of instrument (Stevens 2017). Djembes of different diameters, tubanos, buffalo drums, congas, bongos and hand drums of different sizes and styles are good choices for drum circles.

I try to use one or two bass drums for a drum circle with 15 participants and place the drums in the first circle (in opposite quadrants when using two drums). For larger drum circles, I do not use more than four bass drums, with all the drums placed equidistant from each other in the inner circle. If the bass drums are too close together, then one side of the circle will be louder than the other. This may make it difficult to hear the rhythms and melodies from the higher-pitched drums, and voices singing or giving facilitation instructions. The drums and percussion instruments are put in place around the circle before participants are present so that the instruments and the sounds that are made by them are evenly spread around the circle. Extra percussion instruments and drums are placed on a table outside the circle for participants to select and use at their discretion. Participants are encouraged to select the instrument and seat of their choosing. If a participant brings a personal drum, then that person is encouraged to take a seat in the circle and, if necessary, the surrounding drums will be altered to ensure equality of sound around the circle.

Role of the facilitator

Once the room has been selected and the chairs and instruments have been set out, the drum circle facilitator greets each participant as they arrive. The facilitator should act with humility and provide an open and engaging environment where everyone is welcome and invited to join the drum circle (Ratigan 2009). The definition of facilitator is "somebody who enables a process to happen, especially somebody who encourages people to find their own solutions to problems or tasks" (Encarta 2004, p.664). In a therapeutic drum circle, a facilitator's role would involve creation and maintenance of a therapeutic milieu while supporting and encouraging the participants in the drum circle (Moon 2008). The facilitator will guide the participants and nurture the rhythms of the drum circle, creating an atmosphere of safety, togetherness and enjoyment (Hull 2006).

The facilitator should begin a therapeutic drum circle with a self-introduction and introduce any assistants or staff. This is a good time to ask the group if an intention needs to be set for the drum circle. An intention involves drumming for a purpose and may include symbolic drumming to represent abstract concepts (Lusebrink 1991).

Some drum circles take time to offer an intention for the drum circle prior to drumming. People create an intention or a prayer to drum for any number of things (for example, peace, an ill friend or relative, the good fortune of someone leaving the therapeutic setting). The intention is up to the group, and the facilitator needs to take the lead from the participants to determine whether an intention is needed or wanted. If the participants of the drum group want to drum to symbolize an abstract concept such as peace, this is indicative of functioning at the Symbolic component of the ETC (Hinz 2009; Mank 2019). Functioning at the Symbolic component of the ETC offers the opportunity to develop mastery, self-awareness and transcendence (Hinz 2009).

Throughout the drum circle the facilitator should be attuned to the participants and evaluate the needs of the individual as well as the needs of the group (Knysh 2013). The facilitator should take time to watch each participant to determine the level or component of the ETC in which the participant is functioning (Hinz 2009). The facilitator should also be evaluating for any change in the individual in order to properly determine the next steps to take in facilitation and directives given to the individual and the group.

Social roles and appropriate behavior are modeled by the facilitator throughout the drum circle session and continually from week to week (Mank 2019). The facilitator also displays positive affect and consciously mirrors the behavior and facial expressions of the participants of the group in an effort to activate mirror neurons and build attachment as guided by object relations theory (Kossak 2015).

The facilitator should show unconditional positive regard, or acceptance, of each participant (Rogers 2007). The facilitator initiates exercising unconditional positive regard through the display of enthusiasm, smiling and welcoming the participants to the drum circle group. The facilitator should assure everyone that the drum circle experience is meant for personal growth and healing, which may be achieved through exploration and discovery within the safe environment of the drum circle. The facilitator makes an effort to make and hold eye contact with each member of the group while modeling a positive affect and acceptance for each member of the group, thereby stimulating mirror neurons and beginning to form attunement and attachment (Kossak 2015). The next step should be to educate the participants on how to play the instrument and to practice appropriate drum circle etiquette.

Therapeutic drum circle etiquette

The participants should be asked to remove rings, jewelry and watches to prevent injury to fingers and hands, and damage to the jewelry and drumhead (Wolf 2016). If the participant cannot remove the jewelry, then medical tape to wrap around the jewelry should be offered by the facilitator (Ratigan 2009). If the participant does not want to use tape, then a mallet that can be used to play the drum should be offered instead (Mank, 2019; Ratigan, 2009).The participants should also be informed that the instruments on the table are available for playing and experimentation. If someone leaves the circle, the drum they were playing should not be immediately taken unless it is the only bass drum in the circle. It is important to maintain the pulse of the groove for the benefit of the group. Upon the return of the participant, the drum should be offered back to that participant. Each participant is expected to maintain self-care. If the participant needs a break or needs to change an instrument, then the participant should feel free to do so as often as necessary. Self-care is a vital skill in life and therefore should be respected and practiced in the therapeutic milieu of the drum circle. Most importantly, the group is informed that there is one rule in the drum circle and that is that there are no mistakes. This should reduce anxiety for new participants and act as a way to be open and flexible to creativity and imperfection. The beauty of the improvised drum circle is that rhythm can take everyone, as a cohesive and collaborative group, on a beautiful spontaneous journey full of exploration, creativity and discovery.

How to play a djembe or tubano drum

The drums that are used in drum circles are able to produce different sounds or notes, depending on where and how they are hit (Wolf 2016). Hands or mallets can be used to produce beautiful sounds (Ratigan 2009). The thumb should be lifted above the rest of the hand to avoid hitting it on the drum (it can be quite painful to hit the knuckles of the thumb on the head or rim of the drum). The wrist should be straight and in line with the forearm (Wolf 2016). The arm and hand are held straight and move as one from the elbow. The elbows are held slightly outward from the body for ease of playing (Wolf 2016). The tubano normally has feet and is placed between the legs of the seated player. The djembe can be worn by placing a strap around the waist of the standing player; it can also be played while seated. If the drum is played while seated, the djembe is tipped away from the player to allow the sound vibration to come out of the bottom of the drum. The player wraps their legs around the base of the drum to secure it while playing (Wolf 2016).

The center of the drumhead holds the deepest and richest sound, called the bass or *Gun* (Ratigan 2009; Wolf 2016). The player should hold the fingers together, out straight, and slightly relaxed while hitting the drum with the palm and fingers. The hand and forearm are held parallel to the drumhead and move downward making contact with the drumhead (Wolf 2016). The hand should bounce back off the head of the drum just like jumping on a trampoline (Ratigan 2009; Wolf 2016). A variety of sounds are produced when the hand or mallet is used to hit the drumhead from the center of the drum to the edge. The notes played near the edge of the drumhead are called the tone or *Go* and *Do*, depending on which hand is used (Wolf 2016). *Go* is normally played by the right hand and can be switched if that is not the dominant hand of the player (Wolf 2016). It is higher in pitch than the bass and is played

115

with the pad, knuckles and fingers of the hand. Hold the hands in front of the body with the thumbs and first fingers touching, forming an open triangle. Rotate the hands and arms downward toward the head of the drum. Slide the hands and fingers to the edge of the drumhead until the pad of the palm and knuckles are resting on the rim. The fingers and first knuckles of the hand produce the tone sound, *Go* and *Do*, when hit near the rim of the drumhead. Lift the hand and move the hand downward to make contact with the drumhead. The hand should bounce off the drum as if bouncing on a trampoline and lift straight upward (Ratigan 2009; Wolf 2016).

The slap, or *Pa* and *Ta*, is another sound that is produced from the drum (Wolf 2016). This sound takes practice and can cause injury to the hand for the inexperienced drummer (Ratigan 2009). There are a few ways to produce this sound, which is played on the edge or rim of the drum. I was taught to open my fingers and to hit the pad, or first knuckle of the hand, on the rim at an angle, with fingers spaced apart from one another. The hand should bounce off the drum and move upward (Wolf 2016). Since everyone's hands are different there are several ways to produce sound on the drum, especially the slap, and all require some practice to emit a rich sound that represents self (Ratigan 2009). The slap is not recommended to be taught in the drum circle because of the risk of possible injury for novice drummers (Ratigan 2009).

Therapeutic drum circle warm ups

The culture of the therapeutic drum circle includes active work to provide a safe and therapeutic environment (Ratigan 2009). If the participant is new to the drum circle, a few minutes are taken to inform the participant about the drum selected and how to effectively play it prior to the start of the session. The participant is shown where extra instruments are stored in case there is a desire to try a new instrument. The participant is offered time to ask any questions and most of all, the participant is told how appreciated they are for coming to drum with the community with authenticity and empathy (Donovan 2015; Ratigan 2009).

Often, participants will continue to experiment with the instrument and the group will spontaneously begin to drum and play on their own.

During this time, the facilitator should actively observe the group to identify beginners and to determine at what level, pole or component of the ETC each participant is functioning (Hinz 2009; Lusebrink 2016; Mank 2019). A few minutes are allowed for continued play before the facilitator temporarily stops the group drumming.

Once the group is stopped, the facilitator conducts or continues an introduction that welcomes the group and states the purpose of the drum circle (Donovan 2015). This is to set the unconditional welcoming atmosphere and to reduce the anxiety of new players, thereby curtailing the possibility of resistance developing in the participants (Donovan 2015). A few minutes are taken to properly stretch the body in order to prevent injury (Mank 2019; Wolf 2016). Mank (2019) utilized singing and movement to the folk song "The Hokey Pokey," as a physical warm up to reduce the risk of drumming injuries. Wolf (2016) advises specific movements that stretch muscles and prepare the body for drumming, movement and dance. Consultation with a doctor and obtaining medical approval or clearance prior to beginning any exercise program is always recommended.

Stretching the shoulders, arms, wrists and hands is important to reduce the risk of injury, especially when working with older adults. Roll the shoulders slowly forward while rotating the arms and palms outward, then continue to roll the shoulders upward toward one's ears (Wolf 2016). Once the shoulders are at the highest point, begin to rotate the arms and palms back inward while the shoulder move backward and downward in the shoulder roll. If this was comfortable, repeat two more times.

Next, lift the right arm to shoulder height, if possible. Move the right arm across the body until it extends beyond the left side (Silversneakers 2019). Take the left hand and place it on the upper right arm, slightly above the elbow. Gently press the right arm closer to the body with the left hand and hold in a stretch for 10–15 seconds. The goal is to stretch the arms and shoulders and not to cause pain. If comfortable, repeat the stretch. Then do the same on the left side by crossing the body with the left arm, at shoulder height, and using the right hand to gently push the left arm closer to the body (Silversneakers 2019). Again, if it was comfortable, repeat the stretch.

Now with arms stretched out at shoulder height and elbows straight, rotate the wrists clockwise eight times and then counterclockwise for ten rotations (Kerr 2016; Wolf 2016). The next stretch involves the hands. Make a fist and then stretch the fingers out and apart, then relax the fingers to a loose fist (Kerr 2016). Do that 3–5 times. When finished, shake the hands and arms for a few seconds (Healthline 2019).

With the elbow straight, lift the right arm up until it is parallel to the floor (Redboxfitness 2019; Upliftingmobility 2019). Keeping the elbow straight, lift the right hand up in the universal stop signal. Take the left hand and place the fingers of the left hand perpendicular to the fingers of the right hand (Mayoclinic 2019; Redboxfitness 2019). The palms should face each other. Gently pull the fingers of the right hand back toward the body, stretching the wrist and fingers. Hold this position for ten seconds. Release the right hand and lower the right fingers downward (Mayoclinic 2019; Redboxfitness 2019; Soundfly 2019). Place the fingers of the left hand on top of the right hand, with the left palm side to the back of the right hand's fingers. Gently press the fingers toward the body, keeping the right elbow straight. Hold this position for ten seconds. Gently shake the hands for a few seconds, as if shaking off water from the fingers (HSST 2017). It is recommended that the above stretches are also done after drumming.

If dancing is expected or possible, stretching of the legs is required. It is not always obvious that a person has a physical disability. To reduce a sense of exclusion, chair exercises are recommended to warm up the legs, buttocks and lower back. The participants should be instructed to sit up tall in their chair, drawing in the abdominal muscles with the legs hip-width apart. The participants should then lift their toes off the floor, keeping their heels on the floor, and then lower their toes back to the floor. This should be done seven more times (Kerr 2016; Silversneakers 2019). Once that exercise is over, the participants should be instructed to keep their toes on the floor while lifting their heels a few inches off the floor, and then to lower their heels to the floor again. This should be done eight times (Kerr 2016; Silversneakers 2019).

Rotating the ankles comes next (Eldergym 2019a). Slightly lift the right knee and slowly rotate the foot to the right in a clockwise fashion, completing a circle with the foot. Do eight rotations clockwise and then rotate eight times counterclockwise. Put the right foot down and repeat on the left side (Eldergym 2019a).

Beginning with the right leg, lift the right foot up, in front of the body, until the knee is straight and then bend the knee and lower the foot to the floor (Eldergym 2019b; Kerr 2016). Repeat this exercise seven more times. Now repeat eight times on the left side (Eldergym 2019b; Kerr 2016).

The next exercise requires good, straight posture, with the individual sitting tall in the chair while drawing in the abdominal muscles (Eldergym 2019c; Kerr 2016). The legs should be hip-width apart. Lift the right leg, with the knee bent, a few inches off the chair seat. Repeat seven times (Eldergym 2019c; Kerr 2016). Repeat eight times on the left side. There are more exercises or stretches that can be completed prior to dancing and playing the drum. However, without knowing the physical ability of the participants of the group, it is recommended just to complete the above stretches and allow extra time if someone needs to do any additional stretches that do not take considerable time from the group.

Once the group has been welcomed, has stretched and has been instructed on drum circle etiquette, participants should take a few minutes to connect to the drum and become present in the room (Mank 2019). It is often helpful to take a few relaxation breaths. This involves breathing in through the nose for a count of four, holding the breath for a count of four, and then slowly exhaling through the mouth for a count of eight (Kerr 2016). During relaxation breathing the participants are instructed to inhale positive thoughts such as peace, love or tranquility. On the exhaled breath, the participants are instructed to exhale anything negative or unwanted, such as anger, pain, frustration or worry. The facilitator should give instructions for the first two breath cycles and then give time for several more breath cycles to be completed by the participants without instruction. The participants should then be invited to connect to the drum visually and through touch for two minutes (Mank 2019). The participants should be informed that if their mind wanders, it is natural and they should just refocus on the drum. The facilitator keeps track of the time and counts backward from four to one after the two minutes are up. The facilitator could say, "It's time to come back to this space now. I will count backwards from four to one. You may feel refreshed and connected to the drum. Four, you are coming back to this moment. Three, you are noticing the sounds of the room. Two, you feel your feet on the floor and your body in the chair. One, you are in this present moment and you may feel refreshed and connected." The practice of relaxation breathing and focusing on the drum is to develop presence with, and connection to, the drum as a transitional object while releasing tension and stress from one's daily life and struggles (Mank 2019).

Drum circle directives

There are several ways to facilitate a drum circle. In order to do this, one must be familiar with several basic skills that will aid in entrainment, community building and enable one to start or stop the drumming. It is up to the facilitator to identify what is needed in the moment and how the directive will reach the determined goal. The basic directives listed below are just a beginning; with creativity they can be modified to address the needs of the group, no matter the population or skills of the drummers. Pointing toward people within the drum circle by the facilitator could be considered rude and could negatively affect the development of relationships (Donovan 2015). An open, upward-facing palm directed toward the participant is often better received than a pointed finger and is therefore advised for the following directives (Donovan 2015).

Signaling for attention

The facilitator enters the circle and assumes the orchestration spot. This is often in the center of the circle, depending on the space of the room or location (Hull 2006; Knysh 2013; Stevens 2017). Then the facilitator raises one hand above their head while turning slowly around the circle and making eye contact with the participants. This is done to notify the group that something is about to happen and their attention is needed (Hull 2006; Knysh 2013; Stevens 2017). The facilitator could also walk around the circle with an arm raised and the index finger extended while making eye contact with the group. Once the facilitator has traversed the circle and has the attention of the group, the facilitation directive can commence.

Starting a drum circle

It is important to learn how to start a drum circle. It is recommended one conducts a drum circle with a 4/4-time signature and rhythm structure for novice drummers, although with care a 6/8-time rhythm can be introduced (Hull 2006). A time signature indicates the structure of a rhythm (Coppenbarger 2014; Hull 2006). The numbers in a time signature are stacked on top of one another, much like a fraction. The top number tells the reader how many beats or pulses there are per measure. In the case of the 4/4-time signature, there are four beats or pulses per measure. The bottom number refers to the type of note that represents one beat. In this case the bottom four indicates that the quarter note gets one beat. Within a 4/4 time signature there are four beats per measure and the quarter note represents one beat (Coppenbarger 2014; Wolf 2016).

The instructions for beginning to play, also known as "call to groove," (Hull 2006, p.52) begin with telegraphing the tempo by stepping to the desired beat prior to starting the group or even playing a note (Knysh 2013). The facilitator can then make a variety of statements to signal the call to start playing. For example, "One, two let's all play" (Hull 2006, p.52). Knysh (2013) recommends "One, two everybody play" (p.33). As long as the term fits the 4/4-time signature, the words can vary. Gardstrom (2014) starts an improvised musical session with "One, two, ready play" (p.85). I often say, "One, two, let's have fun," "One, two, play the drum" or "One, two, here we go." I especially enjoy saying that last expression as I think that drum call taps into everyone's sense of adventure since we never really know just where the rhythm will lead us.

Stopping play

Hull (2006, p.55) uses the phrase "stop cut" to stop the group on the first note of a measure. To stop a participant, a subset of the group or the entire group, the facilitator counts backward from four to one and then adds the words "and stop" so that the group stops on the first beat of the next measure (Hull 2006; Knysh 2013; Stevens 2017). The hand and body motions include raising one hand above the head and using the fingers to count down from four to one; then, with a slight hop, cross both hands in front of the body and next swing the arms out to the side, much like a baseball umpire motioning the safe symbol, while the selected group or individuals stop drumming (Hull 2006; Knysh 2013; Stevens 2017).

Keep playing

There are times when the facilitator may want to highlight a few people in the drum circle or may want to facilitate only part of the group. In order to do so, the facilitator must stop some players while others continue to play instruments (Hull 2006; Knysh 2013; Stevens 2017). The facilitator can ask specific people to keep playing via voice or use a hand signal in front of the body. The facilitator bends the elbows outward, with the fingers of one hand pointing toward the elbow of the other arm, and with one hand above the other in front of the body. Then the facilitator circles the hands up and away from the body and then downward and towards the body in a circle (Hull 2006; Knysh 2013; Stevens 2017). The signal is similar to the basketball signal for traveling. Once the participants are selected to keep playing, the rest of the group can be stopped with the signal for stopping play, stop cut (Hull 2006).

Volume

The drum circle group may need encouragement to play loud enough to be heard. At other times the group may need to turn down the volume. The facilitator extends their arms out from the body with hands near waist height, using the palms to indicate the desired direction of volume (Hull 2006; Knysh 2013; Stevens 2017). The facilitator raises their arms with palms up to increase the volume, bringing them overhead if maximum volume is desired. To reduce the volume of the group, the facilitator extends their arms with palms facing downward and brings the hands down slightly toward the sides of the body and toward the floor. The facilitator could also bend their knees and get lower to the ground to signify a low volume or soft sound (Hull 2006; Knysh 2013; Stevens 2017). Changing volume adds dynamics to the song, thereby creating interest within the group.

Sectioning

Large or small sections of the circle can be selected to do something different than the rest of the group (Hull 2006; Knysh 2013). Instead of picking people out individually, the facilitator makes eye contact with the participants and stretches out an arm with the thumb facing upward, bending the elbow and then straightening the arm in a chopping motion to display the edge of the section. The facilitator will then indicate the other side of the section in the same manner. Spreading arms outward toward the edges of the selected section, the facilitator moves their arms toward each other, meeting directly in front of the body. The section is then given directive instructions (Hull 2006; Knysh 2013).

Rocking the boat

This directive begins, as all directives do, with an attention call, and then the facilitator sections the circle into two subgroups. The facilitator stands in the center of the circle, straddling the imaginary line that divides the group into two, with arms outstretched. Each subgroup changes volume in response to the raising or lowering of the arm of the facilitator that is directing the subgroup. The two groups can alternate playing loudly and softly depending on the signals given by the facilitator. In other words, when Subgroup A of the drum circle is playing at high volume, then Subgroup B will be playing at a different volume and often at a low volume so that there is a noticeable contrast between the subgroups. The facilitator effectively raises or lowers the volume of the opposite sides of the imaginary boat, thereby rocking the boat through volume. Hull (2006) uses the metaphor of a teeter-totter to describe this directive. I prefer a boat metaphor, as the differences in volume between the subgroups can be slight or extreme and symbolize the life challenges experienced by individuals of the various populations served within a therapeutic drum circle. The boat metaphor may provide insight into one's own need for a support system and build attachment to the other participants of the drum circle group. A greater sense of attachment is possible when participants become aware of how they are supported by all members of the group to keep the "boat" from capsizing. The facilitator can bring both sides to a matching volume with arms stretched out evenly to the sides and stop the group as a whole.

Sculpting the group

To create an appreciation of the song being created by the group, certain participants can be selected to keep playing while the rest of the group is stopped (Hull 2006; Knysh 2013; Stevens 2017). The participants can be selected by ability, instrument, location in the circle, or other commonalities between the participants. If the group is playing the drums with a symbol of self on it, the participants can be selected by commonalities between the symbols on the drum (Mank 2019). For instance, the facilitator could ask all of the participants with a bird on the drum to continue to play. All the participants with similarities between the drums, which are used as transitional objects, are now identified and play together. This acts as a way to create rhythmic dialog and to initiate attachments between participants of the group (Mank 2019).

The participants selected to keep playing continue to play while the rest of the group, through facial expression, vocals and applause, shows appreciation (Hull 2006; Knysh 2003; Stevens 2017). The rest of the group can join the group through the call to groove directive or can be layered into the song when it is time for the group to come back together as one (Hull 2006; Knysh 2003; Stevens 2017).

Layering

Layering involves selecting participants via instruments to join the groove (Hull 2006; Knysh 2003). I recommend a diverse selection of instruments that include a drum, a bell, a wooden instrument such as clave or rhythm sticks to begin the rhythm. The rest of the instruments played by the participants of the drum circle can be layered in, based on instrument or any other criteria that may act to form attachment, camaraderie or add to the song being created (Hull 2006; Knysh 2003; Stevens 2017). Layering can also work in reverse to stop the group in a more organic manner than what is created with a stop cut (Hull 2006).

Call and response

This is a directive that can be used with the whole drum circle or with a subgroup of the drum circle that has been stopped while the rest of the group continues to play (Hull 2006, Knysh 2003). The group playing provides a platform that supports the rest of the group through holding the pulse and maintaining the established rhythm (Knysh 2013). The facilitator uses an instrument to create and play a rhythm to the subgroup awaiting instruction, and the subgroup echoes the rhythm back to the facilitator. After a few rounds of call and response, the groups can be reunited with the call to groove (Hull 2006; Knysh 2013).

If using as a whole group directive, the same process is conducted with the facilitator playing a rhythm to the whole group (Donovan 2015; Hull 2006; Knysh 2013; Stevens 2017). The whole group then echoes the rhythm back to the facilitator. When the directive seems complete, the facilitator can initiate the call to start drumming and groove with the group.

Group support

Drumming is a way to tune into the moment and be present without conscious thought (Ratigan 2009). Playing a solo while the rest of the drum circle is silent can be intimidating and lead to self-consciousness and a possible sense of failure. For these reasons, the facilitator can lower the volume of the group and then raise the volume for one person to solo while the rest of the group softly supports the pulse and rhythm without overshadowing the participant playing a solo. After a minute or so, the facilitator can lower the volume of the individual and ask the next person to solo. The facilitator should repeat the process until everyone in the circle has a chance to play for the group while simultaneously being supported through rhythm by the group. This directive acts to build trust, a sense of support by the group, and a sense of secure attachment (Mank 2019).

Conversation

A rhythmic conversation can develop spontaneously in the group or as a directive. Often a participant will drum with the group and be noticed by another member. The participants will begin to communicate through rhythm, with one participant creating a rhythm and another responding with something that complements the original rhythm. This collaborative play creates a conversation.

Another way to create a conversation is for the facilitator to play a simple rhythm, such as beating out the syllables to "pepperoni pizza" with bass notes and tones. The facilitator then gestures with palm up to a participant in the circle to respond with a rhythm that is of their own choosing. When complete, the participant selects another participant to respond. This continues until every participant has had a turn. The participants can return to group drumming with the start drumming or layering signal from the facilitator.

Rumble

A rumble is when the participants of a drum circle play as fast as possible (Hull 2006; Knysh 2013; Stevens 2017). This can be done on an individual basis, by a segment of the group or by the entire drum circle, depending on the needs of the group. The indication for a rumble is for the facilitator to quickly wiggle fingers and hands in front of the body. A drum circle can begin with a rumble. The facilitator can add individuals one by one or by segments of the group until the whole group is rumbling (Knysh 2013). A song or the drum circle session can end with a rumble that increases and decreases in volume repeatedly before stopping. The rumble can be stopped with a stop cut or by stopping individuals or segments of the group in a reverse layering, depending on the creativity of the facilitator and the needs of the group (Hull 2006; Knysh 2013).

Developing reciprocal relationships within the drum circle environment

Once the participants of the group have settled into the space and become present, stretched their bodies and perhaps had a brief amount of drumming, the next step is to learn each other's names in an effort to begin relationship development. The facilitator introduces themselves by saying their own name and how they are feeling in the present moment. The emotion is then transformed into a rhythm of the facilitator's choosing. The group then says the name of the facilitator and plays the rhythm three times. The facilitator can then choose to move clockwise or counterclockwise around the circle, giving each person a chance to say their own name, state a feeling and then create a rhythm to depict that emotion. The group repeats the name and the rhythm three times for each participant in the group. It is wise to tell the group that if the rhythm is complex, the group may not get it exactly and will do the very best to copy the rhythm. That way, creativity is not stifled and anxiety is reduced. In addition, there is no need to be perfect and the one rule of no mistakes is held and modeled.

The purpose of this exercise is to learn names while offering validation and acceptance into the drum circle and therapeutic milieu. Appropriate behavior is modeled and each person is acknowledged and accepted while eye contact is made and a reciprocal relationship is begun (Kossak 2015). If there are more than 15 people in the circle it will take too long to complete learning all the participants' names and so this step can be omitted.

If the group is large and there is not time for learning names, an activity to reduce anxiety and begin to build camaraderie is recommended. This could be through a playful activity of singing a folk song as a group (Mank 2019). Other ideas for beginning drumming and forming a connection include air drumming or actual drumming to an ever-increasing rhythm that is sure to fall apart and end in laughter. Another idea is to start a rhythm of bass, tone, and then the group voicing, "I like…" and then rotating around the circle with each individual person shouting something they like. For instance, the group plays the two notes and the group shouts "I like," then the facilitator shouts something unusual or silly such as "eel." Then the group plays two notes, shouts "I like," and the next person clockwise or counterclockwise to the facilitator shouts what they like. This should continue around the circle, with everyone getting a chance to engage. The goal is to pick something silly to make the group laugh.

Another way to reduce anxiety and build community is to create a rhythm by clapping hands, tapping mallet sticks or tapping legs in a variety of ways (Knysh 2013). Once a rhythm is created and played by the group, the tempo should increase until it falls apart. This directive is symbolic of how rhythms can fall apart without causing anxiety. The participants have also learned a rhythm without realizing it and they may have had fun in the process (Hull 2006; Knysh 2013).

After the names are learned, or as the group advances in skills and cohesion is developing, improvisational drumming may commence or continue. Some drum circles are based in traditional rhythms where sections of the group are taught different parts of a rhythmic pattern that are designed to lock together to form a specific song (Knysh 2013). Within the therapeutic drum circle, the emphasis is on creativity and experimentation, resulting in the group working together to form a song based in improvisation and creativity. Both styles have the potential to form community and serve to build mastery and social roles; they may also prove to be an enjoyable experience for the participants (Hull 2006; Knysh 2013; Mank 2019).

Facilitating the group

After starting the group playing, I play whole bass notes on my drum in the beginning of the drum circle session—nothing fancy, just setting the pulse and leaving lots of space between the notes. While playing this way, I am offering plenty of silence for others to fill in with whatever rhythm they choose to create while initiating a pulse for the group to follow. Silence is important so that the participants can offer something creative and the rhythms can lock into place (Hull 2006, Knysh 2013; Wolf 2016). The sounds of the drum become the voices of the participants, especially if playing the drum as a transitional object that represents self (Winnicott 2005). The facilitator must listen to the voices of the participants in order to attune to their individual needs and to those of the group. Leaving silence so that it can be experienced and others are allowed to have a voice is integral to forming a reciprocal relationship (Hull 2006; Knysh 2013; Kossak 2015; Stevens 2012).

If the participants of the group are hesitant to add to the rhythm, the facilitator can add more notes or play a simple rhythm with which the members may experiment. A good technique is to drum to phrases such as "chicka, chicka, boom" (Knysh 2013). The bass note can be played on the boom, if that seems appropriate. The goal is simply to get the group comfortable with playing. It doesn't matter which notes are played as long as it is consistent and within the character of the pulse. Another phrase could be "I like drum-ming, drum-ming." There are often rests, or quiet spots, within the rhythm so that there is space for creativity in which the group can add to the rhythm when improvising a song (Knysh 2013).

Assessment and attunement within the drum circle

While the participants continue to play, the facilitator can walk around the inside of the circle, making eye contact with each participant to stimulate the mirror neurons and model appropriate behavior (Kossak 2015). While walking around the circle, the facilitator can observe the participants to identify drumming ability and possible ETC functioning (Hinz 2009; Ratigan 2009). The facilitator can stop at the chair of each person within the inner circle and play along with them (Ratigan 2009). This is a way to attune to the client and assess the situation (Hinz 2009; Ratigan 2009). If the facilitator uses this time as a way to play and develop rapport with the participants, the participants may feel supported and safe with the facilitator. In this case, the facilitator becomes the good-enough facilitator and acts as secure base for the participants to use rhythm and the bonding experience of the drum circle to develop secure attachments to the facilitator and the members of the drum circle group (Bowlby 1982; Kossak 2015; Winnicott 2005).

This is a time for building a relationship, or rapport, between the individual members of the group and the facilitator, as well as between the members of the group (Kossak 2015). Therefore, the facilitator should play a simple rhythm in order to encourage the novice drummer to play. The space and silence within the simple rhythm acts to lock into a complex rhythm and offers a means to connect to a participant with more advanced skills in drumming (Knysh 2013). If the goal is to try to attain an altered state of consciousness, then the facilitator should be drumming and facilitating a tempo of 4–4½ beats per second (Flor-Henry *et al.* 2017; Maxfield 1990; Sideroff & Angel 2013).

While playing with the participants of the drum circle in a *quasi* one-to-one situation, the participant's level of functioning on the ETC may become evident (Hinz 2009). It is recommended that using the ETC as an assessment tool should only be conducted by a trained mental health therapist (Hinz 2009).

The Expressive Therapies Continuum and drumming

The ETC is a hierarchical and theoretical framework that categorizes expressive arts experiences into developmental progressions of information processing and artistic representations (Hinz 2009). The art expressions and cognitive processing of stimuli, within the hierarchical framework, range from simple to complex. There are three bipolar levels that represent complementary means of processing information. The fourth level is the Creative level, which can appear on any one of the three bipolar levels through the balance of functioning of both poles (called the Creative transition). The Creative level can also be represented by the synthesis of functionality of all the levels (Hinz 2009). The ETC assists individuals in understanding the stimuli and knowledge gained through body sensations and from the world at large (Hinz 2009).

Kinesthetic/Sensory level of the ETC

As described in Chapter 1, the ETC is a theoretical framework that provides a therapist insight into the possible visual information processing of a client (Hinz 2009). The ETC is detailed here to provide information to the therapist to gain understanding of the participants within the therapeutic drum circle group. There are drum circle directives that may assist the therapist to best serve the participants of the drum circle group to function with creativity.

The Kinesthetic/Sensory level is considered to be the least complex level of the ETC in terms of emotional and cognitive development and processing (Hinz 2009). In human development, information processing begins at a preverbal level through tactile and sensory stimuli. Rhythm, tactile and sensory stimuli provide the information that is processed on the Kinesthetic/Sensory level of the ETC (Hinz 2009). The Kinesthetic component is exemplified by the discharge of energy via spontaneous physical movement or gestures, the execution of a specific activity such as drumming, and movement in reaction to external stimuli (Lusebrink 1991). The Kinesthetic component is identified by the display of divergent levels of energy by an individual (Hinz 2009). The individual may exhibit high levels of energy or very low levels of energy or arousal that are depicted in physical movements and gestures (Hinz 2009; Lusebrink 2016).

The Sensory component of the Kinesthetic/Sensory level accentuates internal and external perceptions and sensations that are experienced through touch or by other forms of media and expressive interaction (Lusebrink 1991). Kinesthetic and sensory experiences hold the potential to access and address sensory-based images and impressions that are below the conscious level of knowledge and understanding. To fully understand the inner sensory experience, it is necessary to amplify those inner sensations through relaxation and exclusion from external stimuli (Lusebrink 1991). During this time, one must fully immerse oneself in the sensory experience without exercising conscious control (Lusebrink 1991).

The amount of time between a stimulus and the response to said stimuli is called the reflective distance. On the Kinesthetic/Sensory level the reflective distance is small (Hinz 2009; Lusebrink 1990, 1991). The components of each bipolar level of the ETC complement one another to provide a balance of functioning. The Kinesthetic component is modified by the Sensory component through a reduction of speed and an increase in expression, whereas the Sensory component is altered by the Kinesthetic component through the external expression and release of the sensory impressions (Lusebrink 1991). Within the environment of a drum circle, the Kinesthetic/Sensory level is distinguished by exploration and experimentation of different instruments and by the sensory responses to the sounds created by the instruments (Lusebrink 1991). The Creative transition point of the Kinesthetic/Sensory level would include appreciating the sound and tactile effects of the musical experience while expending some physical energy that may include some semblance of form by way of establishing an improvised rhythm (Mank 2019).

The Kinesthetic/Sensory level offers specific healing dimensions (Lusebrink 1991; Hinz 2009). The healing dimensions of the Kinesthetic pole include the release of energy and the ability to form rhythm. The Sensory pole offers healing dimensions related to increased awareness of inner sensations, along with a slow rhythm (Lusebrink 1991). The emergent function of each of the levels of the ETC includes aspects of the next and higher level. The emergent function of the Kinesthetic/Sensory level includes perception of forms and images, and expressions of emotions and affect that include a higher level of processing within the brain (Lusebrink 1991; Hinz 2009). Within the context of a drum circle, the emergent function of the Kinesthetic/Sensory level could be represented in the drumming group by establishing and holding a moderate tempo and/or rhythm while the group appears to display a positive affect or sense of enjoyment (Mank 2019).

DRUM CIRCLE DIRECTIVES DESIGNED TO DEVELOP A PULSE
In order to assist in finding form in the drum circle, the facilitator could enter the center of the drum circle and try to help to develop a pulse by

telegraphing the pulse through their own body movement and through sound. The facilitator could use an instrument such as a frame drum and model the pulse through beating the instrument while moving their hips and body to the rhythm of the pulse. The facilitator could also wear a shell or bell anklet while stepping to the beat. The bells or shells create a higher-pitched sound than the drums and act to reinforce the pulse. Patience and creativity are required by the facilitator, along with a dedication to serve the participants of the group (Donovan 2015).

Another directive that may act to assist the group in finding form via establishing a pulse within the improvised music is the stop cut (Hull 2006). The facilitator could do a series of starts and stops to build a sense of a pulse, or driving beat, within the music being created. This can be accomplished by first getting the attention of the group. The facilitator should execute the signal for attention by entering the drum circle and raising a hand above their head in the orchestration point, or by walking around the inside of the circle while making eye contact with the group (Hull 2006). Once the facilitator has the attention of the group, they could begin to execute a stop cut by counting backward from four to one (Hull 2006). The facilitator says, "Four, three, two, one and stop, two, start again," while staying on the beat. The directive is designed to get the whole group to stop on a beat and restart together on a beat in an attempt to begin to set a pulse. This can be done several times in a row. If conducted in a sensitive manner, the group would be unaware of the purpose of the directive and just experience a fun experience of stopping and restarting together as a group.

An approach to assist a participant to expel heightened physical energy is by providing opportunities to solo. The facilitator could ask the individual to keep playing by asking using voice and/or by making a hand signal (Hull 2006; Knysh 2013). Once the individual agrees to continue playing, the facilitator could stop the group from playing and listen to the individual's drumming. Once the individual appears to have expelled the energy, the facilitator can ask the group to play again and watch the individual to see if there has been a change in the display of energy and if the individual can entrain to the pulse of the group. The facilitator could also use group support, soloing a participant while the group plays softly in support. In this situation Kinesthetic energy is expelled while the participant is supported by the group, thereby forming cohesion between participants of the group and possible changes in processing, as depicted in the theoretical framework of the ETC (Hinz 2009; Lusebrink 1991, 2004, 2010, 2016).

If the participant is focused on the tactile properties of the drum or by the auditory and sensory experience, that participant may be functioning on the Sensory pole of the ETC (Hinz 2009; Lusebrink 1991, 2016). The above directives, which focus on finding form through rhythm, may affect changes in processing that result in processing at the Creative transition point of the Kinesthetic/Sensory Level or at a higher level of functioning (Hinz 2009; Lusebrink 1991).

Perceptual/Affective level of the ETC

The Perceptual/Affective level of the ETC is the next complex level within the theoretical, hierarchical framework (Hinz 2009; Lusebrink 1991, 2010, 2016). The Perceptual component of the Perceptual/Affective level addresses the development of forms and boundaries (Lusebrink 1991). The use of form depicts both the inner and outer experiences of the individual. The emphasis of the Perceptual component is on structure and organization. Within music, the Perceptual component involves emphasis on the temporal aspects and the patterns perceived. These patterns are recognizable and represent good gestalts (Lusebrink 1991). A good gestalt represents something that is whole, complete and uncomplicated (Corey 1996; Danet 2004).

The emphasis of the Affective component of the Perceptual/Affective level of the ETC includes emotions and mood (Hinz 2009; Lusebrink 1991, 2016). Art and music are vehicles for the expression, evocation and expansion of moods as processed and expressed through the limbic system of the brain (Lusebrink 1991). The healing dimension of the Perceptual/Affective level involves the organization of stimuli perceived through visual, kinesthetic and auditory means and the nonverbal expression of the stimuli in the form of good gestalts with awareness and conveyance of emotions. The emergent function of the Perceptual component includes enhancement of cognitive awareness and a greater understanding of self. There is also an increase in the ability to verbalize, discern and organize experiences (Hinz 2009). The emergent function of the Affective component is the capability to identify and internalize emotions and symbolic images and determine meaning (Hinz 2009).

DRUM CIRCLE DIRECTIVES FOR GREATER
FORM AND INCREASED AWARENESS

The directives that involve stopping and starting hold potential to form cohesiveness within the group and provide a pulse and sense of rhythm (Hull 2006; Knysh 2013; Mank 2019). Another directive that may provide cohesion within the group and provide an educational rhythmic experience is through call and response (Hull 2006, Knysh 2013). As noted above, either a section of the group or the entire group is stopped and the facilitator then models a rhythm on a cowbell or drum and the participants who are not currently playing then mirror the rhythm back to the facilitator (Hull 2006; Knysh 2013). This directive teaches rhythm without overt instruction, creates boundaries and form through listening and then mirroring, and provides opportunities for success within a supportive group environment (Hull 2006; Knysh 2013; Ratigan 2009).

The group support directive provides an opportunity for the participant to express emotions and exhibit rhythm skills while being supported by the group. The participant can experience form and rhythm through the support of the pulse provided by the group while having the opportunity for self-expression and discovery through the solo based in rhythm. The participant may also develop awareness through the experience of supporting others through rhythm.

Cognitive/Symbolic level of the ETC

The next, and most complex level of visual process is the Cognitive/Symbolic level of the ETC (Hinz 2006; Lusebrink 1991). The Cognitive component involves cognitive processing, concept development and verbal processing, and includes logical thought processes, executive functioning and decision-making along with problem solving and a greater sense of motivation (Lusebrink 1991).

The Symbolic component of the ECT emphasizes metaphor and aspects of self, as expressed in the creative arts (Hinz 2009; Lusebrink 1991; 2016). The Symbolic component and symbols created are composed of a multitude of layers of meaning that are composed of Kinesthetic and Affective components. The Creative transition point is evidenced by a sense of spirituality, intuition and discovery of previously unknown aspects of self (Lusebrink 2016).

The healing function of the Cognitive component includes an improved ability to form general concepts related to the individual's personal experience that may lead to a promotion of insight (Lusebrink 1991). The emergent function of the Cognitive component is problem solving while incorporating creativity and verbalization. The healing function of the Symbolic component involves the determination of personal meaning derived from the symbolic expression (Lusebrink 1991). The emergent function of the Symbolic component includes self-discovery, inner wisdom and greater self-esteem, which lead to a greater sense of personal freedom (Hinz 2009). The reflective distance on the Cognitive/Symbolic level is greater than on the other levels and allows for planning or postponement of decisions and actions (Lusebrink 1991). If the symbolic image or expression holds emotionally disturbing content, then the reflective distance can increase. If the symbolic expression is regressive in nature, the reflective distance decreases and is evidenced by regressive behavior or expression (Lusebrink 1990, 1991).

DRUM CIRCLE DIRECTIVES FOR STRUCTURE AND METAPHOR

If the drum group decides to drum to an intention or to represent an abstract concept such as peace, this is indicative of symbolic drumming and functioning on the Cognitive/Symbolic level (Mank 2019). The drum group has utilized cognitive processing to actively and overtly use rhythm to symbolize an idea or feeling. The Symbolic component highlights metaphor. In this case, drumming to an abstract concept involves a representation of the abstract concept in symbolic form. The symbolic nature of drumming to represent an intention or an abstract contract holds opportunity for expression of meaning that may lead to self-discovery, expression of spirituality and intuition (Lusebrink 1991).

The drum circle directives that overtly work to increase structure and form include call and response, group support and conversation. The directive of call and response provides structure through demonstrating a rhythm for the group to mirror back to the facilitator, as accurately as possible. Thereby teaching rhythms, forming entrainment and temporal structure. Group support provides structure and creativity through moments of self-expression based in rhythm while the group holds entrainment for the individual. Conversation is a directive where one person plays an improvised rhythm and then invites someone to respond to the original rhythm with creativity while retaining temporal structure. The exercise is a metaphor for a verbal conversation while utilizing creativity, rhythm and structure. Each person is allowed an opportunity to respond to the original rhythm while expressing personal emotions through rhythm, with the rest of the group witnessing the experience.

Creative level of the ETC

The Creative level is the integration of the ETC components, within one level or all levels, in a unified and cohesive manner manifesting in creative expression (Hinz 2009; Lusebrink 1990, 1991, 2004, 2010, 2016). The therapist is responsible for recognizing and affirming the creative expression of the participant. Through the affirmation and support of creativity within a therapeutic milieu, the participant can develop the ability to perceive and respond to "inner and outer stimuli" (Lusebrink 1991). The drum circle provides multiple levels of stimuli and opportunities for creative expression through music, movement and the symbols created on the drum (Mank 2019).

DRUM CIRCLE DIRECTIVES FOR CREATIVITY
The Creative level of the ETC can be stimulated through any of the directives described in this chapter. The facilitator has the opportunity to utilize any or all of the directives to build cohesiveness, a sense of belonging and creative expression among the members of the group through rhythm, movement and artistic expression (Mank 2019). The ETC provide a means to assess the level of functioning of the participant in order to determine appropriate steps and directives to assist in developing Creative level functioning (Hinz 2009).

Feedback

In the beginning of a multi-session therapeutic drum circle, breaks are often necessary for self-care of the hands and to address participants' stamina since drumming can be physically challenging (Wolf 2016). Stevens (2012) advocates the importance of silence in the music experience. The facilitator should bring the group to a close through a stop cut or reverse layering directive (Hull 2006, Knysh 2013). Once the group has stopped, the facilitator should hold the space for a minute or two without speaking, while absorbing the energy and experience and modeling the desired behavior with the group (Kossak 2015; Stevens 2012). The silence allows the facilitator and the participants of the drum circle to digest and absorb the musical experience, relax and calm the body, and liberate the mind from cognitive work (Stevens 2012). During the break in drumming, which should occur about halfway through the session, the participants are instructed to shake their arms, hands and fingers while providing feedback to the facilitator and group (HSST 2017).

The role of the facilitator is to provide a safe therapeutic milieu through unconditional acceptance and encouragement that allows for honest feedback from the participants (Benjamin 2018). The facilitator should ask questions to the group to understand what was preferred and what was not. The facilitator should also make inquiries regarding the reasons for each opinion in order to best serve the group and to work toward self-expression, growth and healing. The information provided by the group is important and will assist the facilitator in learning valuable information that may transform the experience into one of therapeutic growth for all involved.

Reentry into drumming

Once feedback has been given, the facilitator should begin to bring the participants back into the mindset of community drumming and connection to the drum. Mank (2019) utilized singing to a folk song known to participants to restart the group. The group would sing the verses and add drumming to parts of the chorus or to its entirety. This was to develop a renewed connection to the drum and the group through the expressive arts of singing and drumming. This is a good time to observe the group to assess the cognitive functioning of the group through the ability to recall the lyrics and melody and to play rhythms. Difficulty with memory recall could indicate a possible processing blockage and an inability to access and function at the Cognitive component of the ETC (Hinz 2009; Lusebrink 1991, 2010, 2016).

Once the song is completed, the facilitator could use a method of layering or call to groove to start the group (Hull 2006; Knysh 2013; Stevens 2017). Rumble to start is also effective to begin drumming (Knysh 2013). Rumble to start involves starting the individuals, sections or the entire group through the rumble directive and then initiating a call to groove. The facilitator has now assessed the group and should be familiar with the participants' drumming and movement abilities along with their possible functioning at specific levels of the ETC. The directives initiated should be based on the feedback from the participants as well as the information gleaned from the facilitator's assessment of functioning (Hinz 2009).

Closing the drum circle session

Therapeutic drum circles within day treatment centers normally last 50–60 minutes. The drum circle should draw to a close approximately ten minutes prior to the scheduled conclusion. The closing of the drum circle could end on a reverse layering to a soft, relaxing tempo and volume, if that is appropriate for the setting and participants. If working with youth who need to attend class or another therapeutic group, this may be the appropriate choice. If working with people who struggle with fatigue, an upbeat tempo and higher volume ending may be more appropriate and could result with participants feeling energized. The facilitator could rock the boat or use a rumble on a faster tempo and higher volume for that population (Mank 2019).

Regardless of how the group ends, there should be time reserved to ask the participants for added feedback on the community drumming experience. This offers a sense of ownership and perceived value for the participants while adding to the knowledge base of the facilitator (Mank 2019). If the group is small, each participant could give feedback on whether their mood changed as a result of the experience. If the group meets regularly, then this feedback can be tracked to determine the level and length of effectiveness of the drumming experience. The group should be thanked and praised for participating in the group.

Once again, the hands should be stretched and the shoulders rolled to ensure proper body mechanics (Wolf 2016). The participants should be reminded of, and invited to, the next drum circle. Dismantling of the drum circle should then take place. Mank (2019) wrote that a sense of belonging resulted from drumming and through assumptions of social roles. If appropriate for the individual and population of the group, helping to put the drums away and setting the room back up for its regular use should be accepted and encouraged (Mank 2019).

Conclusion

In conclusion, the therapeutic drum circle is a place for self-expression and healing that requires a therapeutic milieu beginning with room selection. The participants should be treated with unconditional positive regard and provided with mirroring, attunement and role modeling in order to affect attachment and growth (Benjamin 2018; Kossak 2015; Mank 2019; Rogers 2007). The facilitator works to form rapport with the participants and visually assesses functioning on the levels of the ETC (Hinz 2009; Lusebrink 1991, 2004, 2010, 2016). Through the assessment of functioning, the facilitator can then make adjustments in order for the participants to find Creative level functioning (Hinz 2009; Lusebrink 1991, 2004, 2010, 2016). It is through the therapeutic drum circle that individuals may achieve therapeutic growth and change while actively engaging in creativity (Hinz 2009; Lusebrink 1991, 2004, 2010, 2016; Mank 2019).

Conclusion

Art therapy and drumming offer opportunities for growth and healing while building community and a sense of belonging (Mank 2019). Within the therapeutic environment of the art studio and drum circle, unconditional positive regard and mirroring can build attachment and neuroplasticity that can lead to greater self-esteem and greater cognitive and creative functioning (Hinz 2009; King 2016; Kossak 2015; Lusebrink 2004, 2016). The role of the art therapist is multifold and begins with accepting and caring for the client in addition to tending to the art (Allen 1995; Rogers 2007). The art therapist must exercise unconditional positive regard to both the client and the art in a manner that includes being present to and in the therapeutic space and moment, and being open, willing and able to create art alongside the client, while modeling support and value of the client and the artwork created in the therapeutic space (Allen 1995; Rogers 2007).

Research has provided evidence that there is a mind–body connection that is influenced by the art making experience (Malchiodi 2012). The mind–body connection relates to the effects that the mind has on the overall health of the body (Malchiodi 2012). Belkofer and Konopka (2008) found that there were measurable changes in activity of the temporal lobe as a result of art making. The temporal lobe is associated with memories that contain emotional states and content. The mind and body are stimulated in response to the creation or viewing of art, providing evidence that art making is the mechanism of change within art therapy (Belkofer & Konopka 2008).

Art is focused on creations, whereas art therapy is grounded in service and healing (Broderick 2011). Art making within the context of the art therapy process holds potential to stimulate specific areas and exercise alternative pathways of the brain, thereby building neuroplasticity through the formation of new neurons and neural connections (Hass-Cohen & Findlay 2015; Hinz 2009; King 2016; Lusebrink 2004, 2016). The ETC is a theoretical and hierarchical framework that presents a visual representation of the processing of information and stimuli of an individual (Hinz 2009; Lusebrink 2010, 2016). The art holds the capability to contain and evoke deep emotional content. Conceptualizing the art activity and processes through the theoretical framework of the ETC allows the art therapist to identify strengths and blockages in the processing of information across and between levels of the ETC (Hinz 2009; Lusebrink 2004, 2010, 2016).

Object relations theory evolved from Freud's psychoanalysis work. Within object relations theory, the role of the therapist is one of support for the client through the selection and manipulation of art materials, understanding of the symbolic meaning contained within the art image, and the facilitation of a safe and controlled therapeutic space. The therapist and the therapeutic milieu allow for the expression of emotions in a controlled manner that should not overwhelm the client (Kramer 1972; Naumburg 1973; Rubin 1987). Object relations theory, in conjunction with attachment theory, offers opportunities for identifying and restructuring pathological behavior and methods of coping by way of the therapeutic alliance. Art therapy and drumming with a therapist also provide the structure and alliance to form attachment and a sense of belonging (Bowlby 1982; Gillath *et al.* 2009; Kossak 2015; Mank 2019; Rogers 1993; Schaverien 1992; Winnicott 2005). The transitional space and object within the drumming group with a self-ascribed drum, along with the therapeutic alliance, provide participants with the opportunity to play, explore and work toward growth and change (Winnicott 2005).

Art making is evident cross culturally and throughout the ages (Dissanayake 1995). The purpose and latent meaning of ancient art may not be concretely known. However, the fact that it was created, preserved and used in rituals indicates that the art and symbols held meaning for those who created and viewed the art (Dissanayake 1995). Haslam (1997) noted that the art addressed a need and held meaning for the society in which the art was created. The visual arts are transformative and the latent meaning evolves in relation to the needs of the culture or society (Haslam 1997).

The spiritual practices of early humans suggest that they had the capacity for abstract thought, were conscious of temporal and spatial processes, and were able to communicate prior to the development of a formal verbal language (Haslam 1997). Langer (1957) noted that the human mind is active in the construction of thoughts and ideas. The use of symbols to represent deeper meaning is indicative of abstract thought and an intelligent mind. The distinguishing feature between humans and all other living species on Earth is the ability to create and utilize symbols (Wilson 1985).

A sign is something that affirms the existence of an object, experience or occasion across time (Langer 1957). A sign is a representation of something specific and does not hold or convey deeper meaning (Morrell 2011; Wilson 1985). The understanding and use of signs was the origin of the outward expression of the active mind of man (Langer 1957). Symbols and symbolic meaning evolved from man's utilization of signs. Symbols contain and convey abstract thoughts, ideas or concepts. Speech and language are examples of symbols as they are used to communicate concepts and convey meaning (Langer 1957). The essence of humanity is founded upon man's ability to make and convey meaning through symbols, thereby initiating the ability to communicate between fellow human beings (Isserow 2013).

Jung and von Franz (1964) define a symbol as something that suggests deeper meaning than what is initially known. Art images are symbolic and convey greater meaning that what is overtly shown in the visual representation. Man creates symbols as a means to represent concepts and ideas that are not fully understood (Jung & von Franz 1964). The dynamic force of the content contained within the symbol provides potential for connection on an interpersonal and intrapersonal level (Isserow 2013). The symbol, or art image, may hold complex meaning and provide alternative perspectives for the viewer of the image. The emotional connection between the viewer and the art image forms a unification of sorts and binds the viewer to the symbol (Haslam 1997).

The sense of unity between the art image and the viewer is dependent upon the unconscious material held within the symbolism contained in the image (Haslam 1997). Therapeutic growth and change are the result of the communal experience between the symbolic meaning and the viewer (Isserow 2013). The symbol contains meaning that may be unknown on a conscious level. Meaning through the viewing of the image is a mechanism of change and the opportunity for therapeutic growth (Haslam 1997).

As with art, music has been a fundamental component in the daily life and rituals associated with humans (Bittman *et al.* 2001; Cook & British Museum 2013). Improvisational music and drumming provide therapeutic benefits to humans through improvement of mood, a sense of belonging and a reduction of the normal stress response (Bittman *et al.* 2001; Faulkner 2012). Music is prominent in the development of a sense of self and is considered to be an agent of change (DeNora 2000; Rolvsjord & Stige 2015). Music conveys the values of a culture, is influential in expressing emotions, personal and sociocultural identity, and can act as a unification mechanism of a community (Bensimon *et al.* 2008; DeNora 2000; Wanjala & Kebaya 2016).

Music provides a means to achieve an altered state of consciousness, and connection to the collective unconscious and to previously unknown aspects of self (Jung 1963; Rugenstein 2000). Through music, therapeutic change and growth are possible. Drum circles and the music created therein offer opportunities to stimulate the neural networks of the brain, express emotions and allow for spiritual growth and the installation of meaning (Tomaino 2014).

Drumming provides the means to elevate a ceremony to something greater and to possibly form a connection to the divine (Dissanayake1995; Waring 2007). Self-transcendence and spiritual connection are possible through the drum and the music it creates (Dissanayake 1995; Murrell 2010; Waring 2007).

The self-ascribed drums described within this book hold potential for becoming a legacy object. Through the therapeutic experience of making a symbol of self on the drum, the art therapist may gain awareness of the visual processing of the participant (Hinz 2009; Lusebrink 2010, 2016). Through careful direction by the art therapist, the participant may reach Creative functioning on the ETC.

The therapeutic drum circle is a mechanism and venue for self-expression and healing. It is advised that the participants of the drum circle should be greeted and treated with unconditional positive regard. The therapist, acting as a facilitator, should demonstrate mirroring, attunement and role modeling in order to instill rapport, attachment and possible therapeutic growth (Benjamin 2018; Kossak 2015; Mank 2019; Rogers 2007). The therapist/facilitator visually assesses the participants' functioning on the levels of the ETC (Hinz 2009; Lusebrink 1991, 2004, 2010, 2016). The facilitator is able to make adjustments, based on the information gathered while assessing the participants, in order to assist in movement toward functioning on the Creative level (Hinz 2009; Lusebrink 1991, 2004, 2010, 2016). The therapeutic drum circle allows participants to achieve therapeutic growth and change while actively engaging in creativity (Hinz 2009; Lusebrink 1991, 2004, 2010, 2016; Mank 2019).

The purpose of this book is not to advise anyone to operate outside their scope of practice. Art making in a therapeutic environment may be healing and yet not art therapy. Art therapy is based in a therapeutic alliance between an art therapist and a client (AATA 2020). The transitional object of the drum with a symbol of self offers an individual the opportunity to form attachments with the drum and their fellow participants (Kossak 2015; Mank 2019; Winnicott 2005).

Making music within a drum circle can evoke change. However, in order for music making to be music therapy, a music therapist and a therapeutic relationship between the music therapist and a client are required (AMTA 2019). Creating music within a drum circle can be enjoyable and life-changing through the creation of a sense of belonging and attachments; however, that is not enough to be music therapy (AMTA 2019; Hull 2006; Knysh 2013; Kossak 2015; Mank 2019). Fun and enjoyment are possible through art and music and offer opportunities for positive outcomes.

References

AATA (American Art Therapy Association) (2020) *About art therapy.* Retrieved from www.arttherapy.org on August 3, 2020.

Allen, P. B. (1995) *Art Is a Way of Knowing.* Boston, MA: Shambhala.

AMTA (American Music Therapy Association) (2019) *What is music therapy?* Retrieved from www.musictherapy.org/about/musictherapy on March 20, 2020.

APA (American Psychiatric Association) (2013) *Diagnostic and Statistical Manual of Mental Disorders : DSM-5.* Arlington, VA: American Psychiatric Association.

Archibald, L., Dewar, J., Reid, C. & Stevens, V. (2010) 'Rights of restoration: Aboriginal peoples, creative arts and healing.' *Canadian Art Therapy Association Journal 23*(2), 2–17.

Barash, J. A. (2008) *The Symbolic Construction of Reality: The Legacy of Ernst Cassirer.* Chicago, IL: University of Chicago Press.

Baumann, A. E. (2007) 'Stigmatization, social distance and exclusion because of mental illness: The individual with mental illness as a "stranger".' *International Review of Psychiatry 19*(2), 131–135.

Baylin, J. & Hughes, D.A. (2016) *The Neurobiology of Attachment-Focused Therapy: Enhancing Connection and Trust in the Treatment of Children and Adolescents.* New York, NY: W. W. Norton & Company.

Belkofer, C. M. & Konopka, L. M. (2008) 'Conducting art therapy research using quantitative EEG measures.' *Art Therapy 25*(2), 56–63.

Benjamin, E. (2018) 'The creative artists support group: A therapeutic environment to promote creativity and mental health through person-centered facilitation.' *Person-Centered & Experiential Psychotherapies 17*(2), 111–131.

Bensimon, M., Amir, D. & Wolf, Y. (2008) 'Drumming through trauma: Music therapy with post-traumatic soldiers.' *The Arts in Psychotherapy 35*(1), 34–48.

Bienenfeld, D. (2005) *Psychodynamic Theory for Clinicians.* Philadelphia, PA: Wolters Kluwer. Retrieved from https://public.ebookcentral.proquest.com/choice/publicfullrecord.aspx?p=3418328 on April 30, 2020.

Bittman, B., Berk, L., Felten, D., Westengard, J. *et al.* (2001) 'Composite effects of group drumming music therapy on modulation of neuroendocrine-immune parameters in normal subjects.' *Alternative Therapies in Health and Medicine 7*(1), 38–47.

Block, D., Harris, T. & Laing, S. (2005) 'Open Studio Process as a model of social action: A program for at-risk youth.' *Art Therapy 22*(1), 32–38.

Boccia, M., Piccardi, L., Palermo, L., Nori, R. & Palmiero, M. (2015) 'Where do bright ideas occur in our brain? Meta-analytic evidence from neuroimaging studies of domain-specific creativity.' *Frontiers in Psychology 6*, 1195.

Bowlby, J. (1982) *Attachment and Loss. Vol. 1–2.* (2nd ed.). Harmondsworth: Penguin.

Bradley, J. M. & Cafferty, T. (2001) 'Attachment among older adults: Current issues and directions for future research.' *Attachment & Human Development 3*(2), 200–221.

Bretherton, I. (1992) 'The origins of attachment theory: John Bowlby and Mary Ainsworth.' *Developmental Psychology 28*, 759–775.

Broderick, S. (2011) 'Arts practices in unreasonable doubt? Reflections on understandings of arts practices in healthcare contexts.' *Arts & Health 3*(2), 95–109.

Bruscia, K. E. (2014) *Defining Music Therapy.* Gilsum, NH: Barcelona Publishers.

Bucciarelli, A. (2016) 'Art therapy: A transdisciplinary approach.' *Art Therapy 33*(3), 151–155.

Burns, D. D. (1980) *Feeling Good : The New Mood Therapy.* New York, NY: Morrow.

Chapman, L. (2014) *Neurobiologically Informed Trauma Therapy with Children and Adolescents: Understanding Mechanisms of Change.* New York, NY: W. W. Norton & Company.

Chapman, L. M., Morabito, D., Ladakakos, C., Schreier, H. & Knudson, M. M. (2001) 'The effectiveness of art therapy interventions in reducing post traumatic stress disorder (PTSD) symptoms in pediatric trauma patients.' *Art Therapy 18*(2), 100–104.

Cinoglu, H. & Arikan, Y. (2012) 'Self, identity and identity formation: From the perspectives of three major theories.' *International Journal of Human Sciences 9*(2), 1114–1131.

Cook, J. & British Museum (2013) *Ice Age Art: The Arrival of the Modern Mind.* London: British Museum Press.

Coppenbarger, B. (2014) *Music Theory Secrets: 94 Strategies for the Starting Musician.* Lanham, MD: Rowman & Littlefield.

Corey, G. (1996) *Theory and Practice of Counseling and Psychotherapy.* Pacific Grove, CA: Brooks/Cole.

Cormier, R. (2019) *Drumcircles: Guidelines and Tips.* Retrieved from http://synthrick. tripod.com/id31.html on March 20, 2020.

Crumbaugh, J. C. & Maholick, L. T. (1964) 'An experimental study in existentialism: The psychometric approach to Frankl's concept of noogenic neurosis.' *Journal of Clinical Psychology 20*, 585–596.

Danet, B. (2004) '"If you have a lot of clutter it messes up the popup": The pursuit of good gestalts in an online folk art.' *Textile: The Journal of Cloth & Culture 2*(3), 226.

Darnley-Smith, R. & Patey, H. M. (2003) *Music Therapy.* London: Sage Publications.

De Botton, A. & Armstrong, J. (2013) *Art as Therapy.* Retrieved from https://ndnu. on.worldcat.org/oclc/860#870341 on April 30, 2020.

Dean, M. (2012) *The Drum: A History.* Lanham, MD: Scarecrow Press.

DeNora, T. (2000) *Music in Everyday Life.* Cambridge: Cambridge University Press.

Dickerson, D., Robichaud, F., Teruya, C., Nagaran, K. & Yi, H. (2012) 'Utilizing drumming for American Indians/Alaska Natives with substance use disorders: A focus group study.' *The American Journal of Drug and Alcohol Abuse 38*(5), 505–510.

Dickerson, D. L., Venner, K. L., Duran, B., Annon, J. J., Hale, B. & Funmaker, G. (2014) 'Drum-Assisted Recovery Therapy for Native Americans (DARTNA): Results from a pretest and focus groups.' *American Indian and Alaska Native Mental Health Research 21*(1), 35–58.

Dissanayake, E. (1995) *Homo Aestheticus: Where Art Comes from and Why.* Seattle, WA: University of Washington Press.

Dissanayake, E. (2000) *Art and Intimacy: How the Arts Began.* Seattle, WA: University of Washington Press.

Dixon, A. L. (2007) 'Mattering in the later years: Older adults' experiences of mattering to others, purpose in life, depression, and wellness.' *Adultspan Journal 6*(2), 83–95.

Donovan, J. (2015) *Drum Circle Leadership: Learn to Lead Transformational Drum Circles*. Jim Donovan Music.

Edwards, M. (1987) 'Jungian Analytic Art Therapy.' In Rubin, J. A. (Ed.) *Approaches to Art Therapy: Theory and Technique*. New York, NY: Brunne/Mazel.

Eldergym (2019a) *Ankle flexibility exercises for seniors and the elderly*. Retrieved from https://eldergym.com/ankle-flexibility/ankle on March 20, 2020.

Eldergym (2019b) *Knee strengthening exercises for seniors and the elderly*. Retrieved from https://eldergym.com/knee-strengthening-exercises/knee on March 20, 2020.

Eldergym (2019c) *Hip flexor exercises for seniors and the elderly*. Retrieved from https://eldergym.com/hip-flexor on March 20, 2020.

Encarta (2004) *Webster's Dictionary of the English Language* (2nd ed.). New York, NY: Bloomsbury Publishing.

Erikson, E. H. (1963) *Childhood and Society* (2nd ed.). New York, NY: W. W. Norton & Company.

Erkkilä, J., Brabant, O., Saarikallio, S., Ala-Ruona, E. *et al.* (2019) 'Enhancing the efficacy of integrative improvisational music therapy in the treatment of depression: Study protocol for a randomised controlled trial.' *Trials 20*(1). Retrieved from https://ndnu.on.worldcat.org/oclc/8089109670 on March 20, 2020.

Faulkner, S. (2012) 'Drumming up courage.' *Reclaiming Children and Youth 21*(3), 18–22.

Flor-Henry, P., Shapiro, Y., Sombrun, C. & Walla, P. (2017) 'Brain changes during a shamanic trance: Altered modes of consciousness, hemispheric laterality, and systemic psychobiology.' *Cogent Psychology 4*(1). Retrieved from https://ndnu.on.worldcat.org/oclc/7298766002 on March 20, 2020.

Friedman, R. L. (2000) *The Healing Power of the Drum*. Gilsum, NH: White Cliffs Media.

Galligan, A. C. (2000) 'That place where we live: The discovery of self through the creative play experience.' *Journal of Child and Adolescent Psychiatric Nursing 13*(4), 169–176.

Gardstrom, S. (2014) *Music Therapy Improvisation for Groups: Essential Leadership Competencies*. Dallas, TX: Barcelona Publishers.

Germain, A. & Kupfer, D. J. (2008) 'Circadian rhythm disturbances in depression.' *Human Psychopharmacology: Clinical and Experimental 23*(7), 571–585.

Gillath, O., Hart, J., Noftle, E. E. & Stockdale, G. D. (2009) 'Development and validation of a state adult attachment measure (SAAM).' *Journal of Research in Personality 43*(3), 362–373.

Gilroy, A. & McNeilly, G. (2000) *The Changing Shape of Art Therapy: New Developments in Theory and Practice*. London: Jessica Kingsley Publishers.

Goldenberg, I. & Goldenberg, H. (2008) *Family Therapy: An Overview*. Monterey, CA: Brooks/Cole.

Haslam, M. J. (1997) 'Art therapy considered within the tradition of symbolic healing.' *Canadian Art Therapy Association Journal 11*(1), 2–16.

Hass-Cohen, N. & Findlay, J. C. (2015) *Art Therapy and the Neuroscience of Relationships, Creativity, and Resiliency: Skills and Practices*. New York, NY: W. W. Norton & Co.

Hass-Cohen, N., Kim, S. K. & Mangassarian, S. (2015) 'Art mediated intra-interpersonal touch and space: Korean art therapy graduate students' cultural perspectives on sharing attachment based cloth albums.' *The Arts in Psychotherapy 46*, 1–8.

Healthline (2019) *Exercises for treating carpal tunnel*. Retrieved from www.healthline. com/health/carpal-tunnel-wrist-exercises on May 3, 2020.

Hinz, L. D. (2009) *Expressive Therapies Continuum: A Framework for Using Art in Therapy*. New York, NY: Routledge.

Holland, D. C. & Valsiner, J. (1988) 'Cognition, symbols, and Vygotsky's developmental psychology.' *Ethos 16*(3), 247–272.

HSST (Hand Surgery Specialists of Texas) (2017) *Simple exercises to promote strong hands*. Retrieved from https://carpaltunnelpros.com/2017/02/02/simple-exercises-to-promote-strong-hands on August 18, 2020.

Hull, A. (2006) *Drum Circle Facilitation: Building Community through Rhythm*. Santa Cruz, CA: Village Music Circles.

Isserow, J. (2013) 'Between water and words: Reflective self-awareness and symbol formation in art therapy.' *International Journal of Art Therapy 18*(3), 122–131.

Julliard, K. N. & Van Den Heuvel, G. (1999) 'Susanne K. Langer and the foundations of art therapy.' *Art Therapy 16*(3), 112–120.

Jung, C. G. (1963) *Memories, Dreams, Reflections*. New York, NY: Pantheon Books.

Jung, C. G. & von Franz, M.-L. (1964) *Man and his Symbols*. Garden City, NY: Doubleday.

Kaufman, J. C. & Sternberg, R. J. (2007) 'Creativity.' *Change: The Magazine of Higher Learning 39*(4), 55–60.

Kerr, B. A. (2016) *Seated Strength & Flexibility*. Self-published.

King, J. L. (2016) 'Art Therapy: A Brain-Based Profession.' In D. Gussak & M. L. Rosal (Eds.) *Wiley Handbook of Art Therapy*. Retrieved from http://dx.doi. org/10.1002/9781118306543 on March 20, 2020.

Knysh, M. (2013) *Innovative Drum Circles: Beyond Beat into Harmony*. Millville, PA: Rhythmic Connections Publications.

Koc, Z. (2012) 'Determination of older people's level of loneliness.' *Journal of Clinical Nursing 21*(21–22), 3037–3046.

Koffmann, A. & Walters, M. G. (2014) *Introduction to Psychological Theories and Psychotherapy*. Oxford: Oxford University Press.

Kossak, M. (2015) *Attunement in Expressive Arts Therapy: Toward an Understanding of Embodied Empathy*. Springfield, IL: Charles C Thomas.

Kramer, E. (1972) *Art as Therapy with Children*. New York, NY: Schocken Books.

Kramer, E. (2001) 'Sublimation and Art Therapy.' In J. Rubin (ed.) *Approaches to Art Therapy: Theory & Technique*. New York, NY: Routledge.

Kurlowicz, L. (2002) 'Geriatric Depression Scale.' *Medical Surgical Nursing 11*(4), 200.

Langer, S. K. (1957) *Philosophy in a New Key: A Study in the Symbolism of Reason, Rite, and Art*. Cambridge, MA: Harvard University Press.

Levitin, D. J. (2016) *This Is Your Brain on Music: The Science of a Human Obsession*. New York, N.Y.: Dutton.

Lhommée, E., Batir, A., Quesada, J-L, Ardouin, C. *et al.* (2014) 'Dopamine and the biology of creativity: Lessons from Parkinson's disease.' *Frontiers in Neurology 5*, 55. DOI: 10.3389/fneur.2014.00055

Lohmann, R. I. (2007) 'Sound of a woman: drums, gender, and myth among the Asabano of Papua New Guinea.' *Material Religion 3*(1), 88–108.

Longhofer, J. & Floersch, J. (1993) 'African drumming and psychiatric rehabilitation.' *Psychosocial Rehabilitation Journal 16*(4), 3–10.

Lusebrink, V. B. (1990) *Imagery and Visual Expression in Therapy*. New York, NY: Plenum Press.

Lusebrink, V. B. (1991) 'A systems oriented approach to the expressive therapies: The Expressive Therapies Continuum.' *The Arts in Psychotherapy 18*(5), 395–403.

Lusebrink, V. B. (2004) 'Art therapy and the brain: An attempt to understand the underlying processes of art expression in therapy.' *Art Therapy 21*(3), 125–135.

Lusebrink, V. B. (2010) 'Assessment and therapeutic application of the Expressive Therapies Continuum: Implications for brain structures and functions.' *Art Therapy 27*(4), 168–177.

Lusebrink, V. B. (2016) 'Expressive Therapies Continuum.' In D. Gussak & M. L. Rosal (Eds.) *Wiley Handbook of Art Therapy.* Retrieved from http://dx.doi.org/10.1002/9781118306543 on March 20, 2020.

Malchiodi, C. (2013) 'Defining art therapy in the 21st century.' Retrieved from www.psychologytoday.com/us/blog/arts-and-health/201304/defining-art-therapy-in-the-21st-century on May 5, 2020.

Malchiodi, C. A. (2012) *Handbook of Art Therapy.* New York, NY: Guilford Press.

Mank, D. (2019) *Art and drumming: A study on affect, attachment and self-esteem within the older adult population* (doctoral dissertation). Notre Dame de Namur University. Retrieved from https://search.proquest.com/openview/2faf7910aa6a0be88f3d289e32959eee/1?pq-origsite=gscholar&cbl=18750&diss=y on May 5, 2020.

Maxfield, M. C. (1990) *Effects of rhythmic drumming on EEG and subjective experience.* (doctoral dissertation). Institute of Transpersonal Psychology. Retrieved from https://search.proquest.com/docview/303885457 on May 5, 2020.

Mayoclinic (2019) *Forearm stretches for the workplace.* Retrieved from www.mayoclinic.org/healthy-lifestyle/adult-health/multimedia/forearm-stretches/vid-20084698 on March 20, 2020.

McCaffrey Irish World Academy (2013) 'Music therapists' experience of self in clinical improvisation in music therapy: A phenomenological investigation.' *The Arts in Psychotherapy 40*(3), 306–311.

McCarthy, S. (2016) 'Student research: The therapeutic power of music.' *Journal of the Australian Traditional Medicine Society 22*(3), 154.

McClellan, E. (2014) 'Undergraduate music education major identity formation in the university music department.' *Action, Criticism, and Theory for Music Education 13*(1), 279–309.

Moon, B. L. (1998) *The Dynamics of Art as Therapy with Adolescents.* Springfield, IL: Charles C. Thomas.

Moon, B. L. (2008) *Introduction to Art Therapy: Faith in the Product.* Springfield, IL: Charles C. Thomas.

Morrell, M. (2011) 'Signs and symbols: Art and language in art therapy.' *Journal of Clinical Art Therapy 1*(1), 25–32.

Murrell, N. S. (2010) *Afro-Caribbean Religions: An Introduction to Their Historical, Cultural, and Sacred Traditions.* Philadelphia, PA: Temple University Press.

Naumburg, M. (1973) *An Introduction to Art Therapy: Studies of the Free Art Expression of Behaviour Problem Children and Adolescents as a Means of Diagnosis and Therapy.* New York, NY: Teachers College Press.

Ogden, P., Pain, C. & Fisher, J. (2006) 'A sensorimotor approach to the treatment of trauma and dissociation.' *The Psychiatric Clinics of North America 29*(1), 263–279.

Paukert, A. L., Pettit, J. W., Kunik, M. E., Wilson, N. *et al.* (2010) 'The roles of social support and self-efficacy in physical health's impact on depressive and anxiety symptoms in older adults.' *Journal of Clinical Psychology in Medical Settings 17*(4), 387–400.

Rappaport, L. (2009) *Focusing-Oriented Art Therapy: Accessing the Body's Wisdom and Creative Intelligence.* London: Jessica Kingsley Publishers.

Ratigan, S. (2009) *A Practical Guide to Hand Drumming and Drum Circles*. Retrieved from https://ndnu.on.worldcat.org/oclc/455462081 on May 3, 2020.

Redboxfitness (2019) *Forearm stretches*. Retrieved from https://redboxfitness.com/forearm-stretches on May 5, 2020.

Richardson, G. E. (2002) 'The metatheory of resilience and resiliency.' *Journal of Clinical Psychology 58*(3), 307–321.

Rise, J., Sheeran, P. & Hukkelberg, S. (2010) 'The role of self-identity in the theory of planned behavior: A meta-analysis.' *Journal of Applied Social Psychology 40*(5), 1085–1105.

Robbins, A. (1987) *The Artist as Therapist*. New York, NY: Human Sciences Press.

Robbins, A. (1998) *Therapeutic Presence: Bridging Expression and Form*. London: Jessica Kingsley Publishers.

Rogers, C. R. (2007) 'The necessary and sufficient conditions of therapeutic personality change.' *Psychotherapy 44*(3), 240–248.

Rogers, N. (1993) *The Creative Connection: Expressive Arts as Healing*. Palo Alto, CA: Science & Behavior Books.

Rolvsjord, R. & Stige, B. (2015) 'Concepts of context in music therapy.' *Nordic Journal of Music Therapy 24*(1), 44–66.

Rubin, J. A. (1987) *Approaches to Art Therapy: Theory and Technique*. New York, NY: Brunner/Mazel.

Rubin, J. A. (2001) *Approaches to Art Therapy: Theory and Technique*. Philadelphia: Brunner-Routledge.

Rubin, J. A. (2016) 'Psychoanalytic Art Therapy.' In D. Gussak & M. L. Rosal (Eds.) *Wiley Handbook of Art Therapy*. Chichester: John Wiley & Sons.

Rugenstein, L. (2000) 'Music as a vehicle for inner exploration: The bonny method of guided imagery and music (GIM).' *Guidance & Counseling 15*(3), 23.

Schaverien, J. (1992) *The Revealing Image: Analytical Art Psychotherapy in Theory and Practice*. London: Tavistock/Routledge.

Schaverien, J. (1999) 'The death of an analysand: Transference, countertransference and desire.' *Journal of Analytical Psychology 44*(1), 3–28.

Schore, A. (2000) 'Attachment and the regulation of the right brain.' *Attachment & Human Development 2*(1), 23–47.

Schore, J. & Schore, A. (2008) 'Modern attachment theory: The central role of affect regulation in development and treatment.' *Clinical Social Work Journal 36*(1), 9–20.

Schulenberg, S. E., Schnetzer, L. W. & Buchanan, E. M. (2011) 'The Purpose in Life Test-Short Form: Development and Psychometric Support.' *Journal of Happiness Studies: An Interdisciplinary Forum on Subjective Well-Being 12*(5), 861–876.

Semenza, D. C. (2018) 'Feeling the beat and feeling better: Musical experience, emotional reflection, and music as a technology of mental health.' *Sociological Inquiry 88*(2), 322–343.

Sideroff, S. & Angel, S. (2013) 'The use of drumming.' *Annals of Psychotherapy & Integrative Health 16*(2), 70.

Silversneakers (2019) *Stretching for seniors: 7 simple moves for the not so flexible*. Retrieved from www.silversneakers.com/blog/stretching-for-seniors-7- simple-moves-for-the- not-so-flexible on May 5, 2020.

Soundfly (2019) *Wrist and hand exercises for drummers*. Retrieved from https://flypaper.soundfly.com/write/wrist-and-hand-exercises-for-drummers on March 22, 2020.

Smith, G. D. (2013) *I Drum, Therefore I Am: Being and Becoming a Drummer*. Burlington, VT: Ashgate.

Stets, J. E. & Burke, P. J. (2000) 'Identity theory and social identity theory.' *Social Psychology Quarterly 63*(3), 224–237.

Stevens, C. (2012) *Music Medicine: The Science and Spirit of Healing Yourself with Sound.* Boulder, CO: Sounds True.

Stevens, C. (2017) *The Art and Heart of Drum Circles* (2nd ed.). Milwaukee, WI: Hal Leonard.

Stott, S. (2017) 'Copying and attunement: The search for creativity in a secure setting.' *International Journal of Art Therapy 23*(1), 45–51.

Thagard, P. & Stewart, T. C. (2011) 'The AHA! experience: Creativity through emergent binding in neural networks.' *Cognitive Science 35*(1), 1–33.

Thomson, P. & Jaque, V. S. (2017) *Creativity and the Performing Artist: Behind the Mask.* London: Academic Press.

Tomaino, C. M. (2014) 'Creativity and improvisation as therapeutic tools within music therapy.' *Annals of New York Academy of Sciences 1303*, 84–86.

Ulman, E. (2001) 'Variations on a Freudian Theme: Three Art Therapy Theorists.' In J. Rubin (Ed.) *Approaches to Art Therapy: Theory and Technique.* New York, NY: Taylor and Francis Group.

Upliftingmobility (2019) *7 senior-friendly hand exercises to combat arthritis.* Retrieved from www.upliftingmobility.com/exercises-combat-arthritis on March 22, 2020.

Van der Kolk, B. A. (2014) *The Body Keeps the Score: Brain, Mind, and Body in the Healing of Trauma.* New York, NY: Penguin Books.

Wanjala, H. & Kebaya, C. (2016) 'Popular music and identity formation among Kenyan youth.' *Muziki 13*(2), 20–35.

Waring, D. (2007) *Making Drums.* New York, NY: Sterling.

Wigram, T. (2004) *Improvisation: Methods and Techniques for Music Therapy Clinicians, Educators and Students.* London: Jessica Kingsley Publishers.

Wilson, L. (1985) 'Symbolism and art therapy: I. Symbolism's role in the development of ego functions.' *American Journal of Art Therapy 23*, 79–88.

Winkelman, M. (2003) Complementary therapy for addiction: "Drumming out drugs". *American Journal of Public Health 93*(4), 647–651.

Winnicott, D. W. (2005) *Playing and Reality.* New York: Routledge.

Wolf, Z. (2016) *Whole Person Drumming: Your Journey into Rhythm.* Port Townsend, WA: Publishing-Partners.

Wright, K. (2009) *Mirroring and Attunement: Self-Realization in Psychoanalysis and Art.* Hove, East Sussex: Routledge.

Index

AATA 19, 20, 36
Ainsworth, Mary 52
Allen, P.B. 12, 22, 23, 24, 36, 61, 65, 140
ambivalence 46–8
AMTA 11, 72, 144
Angel, S. 74, 129
APA 47
archetypes 62–3
Archibald, L. 70
Arikan, Y. 69, 70
Armstrong, J. 41
art making
    in art therapy 22–4
    and Expressive Therapies
        Continuum 31–2
    role of 21–2, 140–1
art therapists
    role of 12
art therapy
    approaches to 19–20
    art making in 22–4
    benefits of 11
    description of 19
    and neuroscience 24–6
    and object relations theory 48–50
    and psychodynamic theory 39–40
    and sublimation 42–3
    symbols in 65
Art Therapy Relational
    Neuroscience (ATR-N) 34–6
attachment theory
    and drumming 56
    and neurological development 53–6
    and psychodynamic theory 51–6

Barash, J.A. 60
Baumann, A.E. 77
Baylin, J. 54
Belkofer, C.M. 25, 140
Benjamin, E. 139, 143
Bensimon, M. 75, 76, 81, 82, 83, 143
Bienenfeld, D. 35, 37, 38, 39
Bittman, B. 80, 81, 143
Block, D. 35
Boccia, M. 76
Bowlby, J. 51, 52, 53, 55, 56, 57, 129, 141
Bradley, J.M. 53
Bretherton, I. 51, 52
British Museum 21, 22, 81, 143
Broderick, S. 12, 36, 140
Bruscia, K.E. 72, 73, 74
Bucciarelli, A. 24
Buchanan, E.M. 14
Burke, P.J. 69, 70
Burns, D.D. 77

Cafferty, T. 51, 53
Chapman, L. 12, 25, 53, 54, 55, 65, 77
Cinoglu, H. 69, 70
Cognitive/Symbolic level of
    ETC 30–1, 107, 134–6
Cook, J. 21, 22, 81, 143
Coppenbarger, B. 121
Corey, G. 13, 44, 45, 46, 47, 48, 133
Cormier, R. 80
countertransference 40–2
CREATE (Creative embodiment,
    Relational resonating, Expressive

communicating, Adaptive
responding, Transformative
integrating and Empathizing
and compassion) 34–6
Creative level of ETC 136
creativity 76–7
Crumbaugh, J.C. 14
culture and symbols 61–2

Danet, B. 133
Darnley-Smith, R. 11, 72, 73, 74
De Botton, A. 41
Dean, M. 82, 84, 85
DeNora, T. 71, 81, 143
Dickerson, D.L. 75, 83, 85
Dissanayake, E. 20, 21, 22, 40,
    41, 44, 58, 66, 70, 82, 83, 84,
    107, 108, 109, 141, 143
division of mind 38–9
Dixon, A.L. 77
djembe drum playing 155–16
Donovan, J. 50, 109, 116, 117, 120, 132
dream imagery 62
drum circles
    assessment in 128–9
    attention signaling 120
    call and response 124–5
    case vignettes 13–17
    closing session 138–9
    conversation in 125–6
    description of 78–9
    and ETC 129–36
    etiquette in 114–15
    facilitator role in 112–14, 128, 143–4
    feedback 136–7
    group support 125
    instrument selection and
        placing 111–12
    keep playing 122
    layering 124
    playing djembe or tubano
        drum 115–16
    purpose of 79–81
    reciprocal relationships in 126–8
    reentry into 137–8
    rocking the boat 123
    room set up 111
    rumble in 126

sculpting group 123–4
sectioning 122–3
starting 120–1
stopping play 121
structure of 109–10
volume 122
warm ups 116–20
drum making
    author's history 85–7
    tubano drum 87–103
DRUMBEAT protocol 79–80
drumming
    and attachment theory 56
    gender in 84–5
    history of 82
    and object relations theory 50–1
    rhythm in 84
    shamanic 74–6
    and spirituality 82–4
    symbols in 65–6

Edwards, M. 60
Eldergym 118, 119
Encarta 113
Erikson, E.H. 92
Erkkilä, J. 76
etiquette in drum circles 114–15
expressive arts and identity 69–71
Expressive Therapies Continuum (ETC)
    and art making 31–2
    in case vignettes 17
    description of 12–13, 26–7
    and drum circles 129–36
    at Cognitive/Symbolic level
        30–1, 107, 134–6
    at Creative level 136
    at Kinesthetic/Sensory level
        27–9, 105–6, 130–3
    and neuroscience 32–4
    at Perceptual/Affective level
        29–30, 106, 133–4
    and symbol of self 104–7

facilitator role in drum circles
    112–14, 128, 143–4
Faulkner, S. 75, 79, 80, 81, 143
Findlay, J.C. 12, 34, 35, 36, 141
Fisher, J. 32

Floersch, J. 75
Flor-Henry, P. 74, 75, 129
Friedman, R.L. 84
Freud, Sigmund 37–9, 48

Galligan, A.C. 77
Gardstrom, S. 77, 78, 121
gender in drumming 84–5
Geriatric Depression Scale (GDS) 14
Germain, A. 84
Gillath, O. 13, 14, 18, 52, 53, 57, 141
Gilroy, A. 41
Goldenberg, H. 13, 44, 46
Goldenberg, I. 13, 44, 46

Harris, T. 35
Haslam, M.J. 58, 59, 61, 63, 64, 142, 143
Hass-Cohen, N. 12, 24, 34, 35, 36, 141
Healthline 118
Hinz, L.D. 12, 13, 17, 18, 26, 27, 28,
    29, 30, 31, 32, 33, 34, 36, 77, 104,
    105, 106, 107–8, 113, 117, 129,
    130, 131, 133, 134, 135, 136, 137,
    138, 139, 140, 141, 143, 144
Holland, D.C. 61–2
HSST 118, 137
Hughes, D.A. 54
Hukkelberg, S. 69–70
Hull, A. 11, 17, 18, 78, 79, 80, 81,
    83, 109, 111, 113, 120, 121,
    122, 123, 124, 125, 126, 127,
    128, 132, 134, 137, 138, 144

identity and expressive arts 69–71
improvisation 77–8
Isserow, J. 60, 142

Jaque, V.S. S76
Julliard, K.N. 64, 65
Jung, C.G. 60, 62, 63, 65, 66,
    71, 81, 107, 142, 143

Kaufman, J.C. 76
Kebaya, C. 11, 70, 72, 81, 143
Kerr, B.A. 118, 119
Kim, S.K. 24
Kinesthetic/Sensory level of
    ETC 27–9, 105–6, 130–3
King, J.L. 12, 26, 140, 141

Knysh, M. 79, 120, 121, 122, 123,
    124, 125, 126, 127, 128, 129,
    132, 134, 137, 138, 144
Koc, Z. 77
Koffmann, A. 37
Konopka, L.M. 25, 140
Kossak, M. 12, 17, 50, 51, 54, 55–6,
    57, 104, 114, 127, 128, 129, 137,
    139, 140, 141, 143, 144
Kramer, E. 13, 42, 43, 57, 103, 141
Kupfer, D.J. 84
Kurlowicz, L. 14

Laing, S. 35
Langer, S.K. 59, 60, 64, 65, 66, 142
Levitin, D. J. 68
Lhommée, E. 76
Lohmann, R.I. 85
Longhofer, J. 75
Lusebrink, V.B. 12, 17, 18, 26, 27, 28, 29,
    30, 31, 32, 33, 34, 36, 105, 106, 107,
    108, 113, 117, 130, 131, 133, 134,
    135, 136, 137, 139, 140, 141, 143, 144

Mahler, Margaret 45
Maholick, L.T. 14
Malchiodi, C. 19, 20, 21, 24, 25, 140
Mangassarian, S. 24
Mank, D. 11, 12, 13, 14, 17, 18, 50,
    51, 53, 56, 57, 65, 66, 75, 79,
    81, 91, 104, 113, 117, 119, 120,
    124, 125, 131, 134, 135, 136,
    137, 138, 139, 141, 143, 144
Maxfield, M.C. 74, 75, 129
Mayoclinic 118
McCaffrey Irish World Academy 69, 72
McCarthy, S. 74
McClellan, E. 69
McNeilly, G. 41
mental health and music 71–2
mirroring 53–6
Moon, B.L. 19, 23, 113
Morrell, M. 59, 142
Murrell, N.S. 83, 108, 143
music
    function of 67–9
    improvisation 77–8
    and mental health 71–2
    and music therapy 72–4
music therapy 72–4

Naumburg, M. 13, 24, 39, 40, 41, 42, 57, 141
neuroplasticity 34–6
neurological development 53–6
neuroscience
    and art therapy 24–6
    and Expressive Therapies Continuum 32–4
    neuroplasticity 34–6
normal infantile autism 45–6

object relations theory
    ambivalence 46–8
    and art therapy 48–50
    description of 13
    and drumming 50–1
    normal infantile autism 45–6
    and psychodynamic theory 44–8
    symbiosis 46
Ogden, P. 32, 33
Olatunji, Babtunde 83

Pain, C. 32
Patey, H.M. 11, 72, 73, 74
Paukert, A.L. 77
Perceptual/Affective level of ETC 29–30, 106, 133–4
psychodynamic theory
    and art therapy 39–40
    attachment theory 51–6
    countertransference 40–2
    division of mind 38–9
    Freud's theories on 37–9
    levels of consciousness 38
    mirroring 53–6
    and object relations theory 44–8
    sublimation 42–3
    transference 40–2
Purpose in Life Test (PIL) 14–15

Rappaport, L. 19, 20, 23
Ratigan, S. 109, 111, 113, 115, 116, 125, 129, 134
Redboxfitness 118
rhythm in drumming 84
Richardson, G.E. 35
Rise, J. 69–70
Robbins, A. 46, 47, 48, 49, 50, 51

Rogers, C.R. 12, 53, 56, 57, 104, 114, 139, 140, 141, 143
Rogers, N. 70
Rolvsjord, R. 71, 143
Rubin, J.A. 13, 38, 39, 40, 42, 57, 60, 61, 141
Rugenstein, L. 71, 81, 84, 143

Schaverien, J. 41, 56, 57, 141
Schnetzer, L. 14
Schore, A. 53, 55
Schore, J. 53
Schulenberg, S.E. 14
Semenza, D.C. 11, 69, 71, 72
shamanic drumming 74–6
Sheeran, P. 69–70
Sideroff, S. 74, 129
Silversneakers 117, 118
Smith, G.D. 85
Soundfly 118
spirituality and drumming 82–4
State Adult Attachment Measure (SAAM) 14, 15
Sternberg, R.J. 76
Stets, J.E. 69, 70
Stevens, C. 11, 18, 50, 72, 79, 80–1, 112, 120, 121, 122, 123, 124, 125, 126, 128, 136, 137, 138
Stewart, T.C. 76
Stige, B. 71, 143
Stott, S. 54, 55
Strange Situation assessment 52
sublimation 42–3
symbiosis 46
symbol of self 104–7
symbols
    archetypes 62–3
    in art therapy 65
    connection to 63–5
    and culture 61–2
    dream imagery 62
    in drumming 65–6
    in history 58–9
    theories of 59–61, 142–3

Thagard, T. 76
Thomson, P. 76
Tomaino, C.M. 76, 81, 143
transference 40–2

tubano drum
  making 87–103
  playing 115–16

Ulman, E. 24, 40
Upliftingmobility 118

Valsiner, J. 61–2
Van Den Heuvel, G. 64, 65
Van der Kolk, B.A. 44, 54
von Franz, M.-L. 60, 62, 63, 66, 142

Walters, M.G. 37
Wanjala, H. 11, 70, 72, 81, 143
Waring, D. 82, 83, 107, 108, 143
warm ups for drum circles 116–20
Wigram, T. 76, 78
Wilson, L. 61, 142
Winkelman, M. 75, 78
Winnicott, D.W. 17, 18, 44, 46, 48,
  49, 50, 51, 53, 54, 55, 56, 57,
  66, 104, 128, 129, 141, 144
Wolf, Z. 83, 115, 116, 117,
  118, 128, 136, 138
Wright, K. 54, 55